# EXTRADIGESTIVE MANIFESTATIONS OF HELICOBACTER PYLORI INFECTION - AN OVERVIEW

Edited by **Bruna Maria Roesler**

**Extradigestive Manifestations of Helicobacter Pylori Infection - An Overview**
http://dx.doi.org/10.5772/60791
Edited by Bruna Maria Roesler

**Contributors**

Ki Baik Hahm, Kyu Hyun Han, Jong-Min Park, Young Min Han, Joo Young Cho, Weon Jin Ko, Sue Kyung Park, Germán Campuzano-Maya, Sebahat Basyigit, Ferdane Sapmaz, Ayse Kefeli, Metin Uzman, Khitam Muhsen, Saeda Haj, Michal Raviv, Natalina Miguel

**Published by InTech**

Janeza Trdine 9, 51000 Rijeka, Croatia



**Publishing Process Manager** Iva Simcic

**Technical Editor** SPi Global

**Cover** InTech Design team

First published July, 2016

Printed in Croatia

Additional hard copies can be obtained from orders@intechopen.com

Extradigestive Manifestations of Helicobacter Pylori Infection - An Overview, Edited by Bruna Maria Roesler

p. cm.

Print ISBN 978-953-51-2461-0
Online ISBN 978-953-51-2462-7

For EU product safety concerns:
IN TECH d.o.o., Prolaz Marije Krucifikse Kozulić 3, 51000 Rijeka, Croatia,
info@intechopen.com or visit our website at intechopen.com.

# Meet the editor

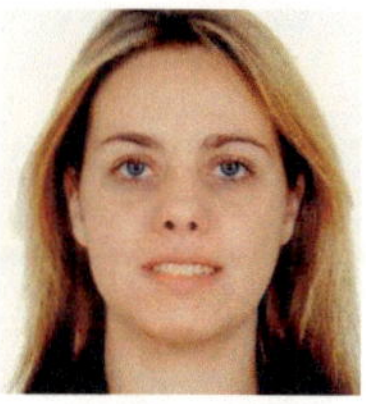

Dr. Bruna Maria Roesler is a pharmacist/biochemist and holds a Master Degree in Pharmacology and a Doctoral Degree in Basic Sciences – Internal Medicine from the State University of Campinas (Campinas, SP, Brazil), where she has identified the principal genotypes of Helicobacter pylori in patients with chronic gastritis, peptic ulcer disease and gastric adenocarcinoma through molecular biology techniques. She has published her work in several peer-reviewed journals and she held presentations at various congresses. She is a member of the Helicobacter pylori Research Group Study from the State University of Campinas, including the study of etiology, epidemiology and physiopathology of gastrointestinal diseases. Her current research includes the study of Helicobacter pylori and pancreas diseases and perigastric lymph nodes from patients with gastric cancer.

# Contents

# Preface

The possible relationship between *Helicobacter pylori (H. pylori)* infection and the development of extragastric disorders still remains a controversial and arguable topic. Different pathogenic mechanisms have been hypothesized, including the induction of a low-grade inflammatory state and the occurrence of molecular mimicry mechanisms. Nevertheless, while some studies are quite large and well conducted, in other cases there are just small or isolated case reports concerning the theme.

*H. pylori,* isolated for the first time in 1983 by Warren and Marshall, is an ancient microorganism that has co-evolved with humans for over 60,000 years and nowadays affects more than half of the world population. *H. pylori* presents well-characterized mechanisms of adaptation, which were developed over the time. Through selection and coevolution, this bacterium established measures by which it actively and passively avoids the human immune response.

*H. pylori* infection is the main cause of chronic gastritis, peptic ulcer disease, mucosa-associated lymphoid tissue (MALT) lymphoma and gastric cancer. In 1994, the International Agency for Research on Cancer (the World Health Organization) classified *H. pylori* as a class I carcinogen because of the epidemiological link of this microorganism infection with a higher risk of development of gastric malignancy.

The infection is typically acquired during childhood and usually becomes a lifelong infection, if left untreated. The host certainly mounts an immune response, but it fails to clear the infection, and *H. pylori*successfully establishes a persistent infection leading to chronic inflammation. Nevertheless, it has been estimated that only 10% of people colonized with this bacterium portray disease symptoms, a fact that suggests that both host and bacterial factors can contribute to differences in *H. pylori* pathogenicity. Besides, it is important to consider that together with the host characteristics and bacterial virulence, the environmental factors also contribute for the clinical outcome of *H. pylori* infections.

Recently, *H. pylori* is increasingly being associated with extragastric diseases, and this association has been reported by several studies which results range from definitive confirmation of the bacterial responsibility in the pathogenesis of some diseases to overall rather controversial results. According to the mentioned studies, this microorganism infection has been associated with hematological diseases, cardiovascular diseases, hepatobiliary and pancreatic diseases, skin and pulmonary diseases, insulin resistance, diabetes and its complications and neurodegenerative disorders, among others.

As regards to hematological diseases, there is substantial evidence in favour of an association between *H. pylori* infection and unexplained iron deficiency anemia, idiopathic thrombocytopenic purpura and vitamin $B_{12}$ deficiency. Considering it, the principal guidelines for the management of *H. pylori* infection recommends that the infection should be sought and treated.

An association between *H. pylori* infection and coronary artery disease as well as with atherosclerosis has been described but remains controversial. In the same way, studies described a link between this microorganism presence and lung diseases, such as chronic obstructive pulmonary disease. Despite of it, there is insufficient evidence to draw conclusions regarding the role of *H. pylori* infection and these disorders.

The same possible association has been described between this infection and hepatobiliary and pancreatic disorders. There are many lines of evidence that *H. pylori*, especially the most virulent strains, can contribute to hepatocellular carcinoma, cirrhosis and chronic hepatitis, as well as to pancreatic cancer and chronic pancreatitis. Notwithstanding, some studies suggest that this pathogen may represent a co-risk factor for these conditions.

Considering the hypothesis and the importance that *H. pylori* isolation and its studies have represented to the scientific and medical communities, this book contemplates very important reviews and studies that highlight our view about the influence or responsibility of this infection in extradigestive disorders. Consequently, this book is compound by seven chapters, which are divided into following sections: General comments on *H. pylori* infection and extradigestive diseases; *H. pylori* infection and oral cavity; Hematological diseases and *H. pylori* infection; and *H. pylori* and metabolic disorders.

**Dr. Kyung Park** presents an interesting chapter regarding important aspects reported to *H. pylori*infection and extragastric diseases. Discussions concerning this infection and dyslipidemia, hypertension, insulin resistance and diabetes, obesity, metabolic syndrome and obesity, atherosclerosis, autoimmune diseases and other extradigestive diseases such as migraine and chronic bronchitis are depicted.

**Prof. Ki Baik Hahm** and colleagues report halitosis as one of extragastric manifestations of *H. pylori*, also considering that Korean red ginseng could be a natural product very effective in relieving halitosis in addition to responsible bacterial suppression.

In the third section of the book, three important chapters describe the relationship between *H. pylori*infection and hematological diseases. **Dr. Campuzano-Maya** described the principal aspects of iron deficiency anemia, vitamin $B_{12}$ deficiency and immune thrombocytopenia, besides other hematological diseases not really associated with *H. pylori* infection, such as immune neutropenia, antiphospholipid syndrome and plasma cell dyscrasias.

**Dr. Miguel** reports the interaction between *H. pylori* and the immune system, describing the principal aspects of iron deficiency anemia, idiopathic thrombocytopenic purpura and MALT lymphoma pathogenesis. Topics concerning the principal mechanisms of pathogenesis as well as the principal diagnostic tests, epidemiology and routes of transmission are also explained.

**Dr. Basyigit** and colleagues present an interesting chapter concerning *H. pylori* and iron deficiency anemia, considering all the important aspects of this disease, including the iron metabolism, possible mechanisms of iron deficiency related to *H. pylori* infection and the management of the disease, among other topics.

Finally, in the last section of this book, **Dr. Muhsen** and colleagues report the principal evidence of the possible relationship between *H. pylori* and diabetes mellitus, including the changes in gastric physiology and metabolic homeostasis, besides the possible rule of bacteria on metabolic syndrome.

"Extradigestive Manifestations of *Helicobacter pylori* – An Overview" will certainly provide an updated set of information in all the principal aspects of this so curious and important relationship, enriching the knowledge of the whole scientific community about this ancient microorganism, which can really be recognized as a "master of adaptation".

The editor dedicates this book to Dr. Zeitune, her advisor who unfortunately passed away in the course of this project. The editor expresses her thankfulness for the excellent work of the contributing authors. The editor thanks Ms. Danijela Duric and Ms. Ana Pantar for all their attention and support, making possible the accomplishment of this book. The editor is especially thankful for the excellent support given by Ms. Iva Simcic in all the steps of this book, as well as the entire InTech Open Access publishing team.

**Dr. Bruna Maria Roesler**
Pharmacist Biochemist
Department of Internal Medicine
Center of Diagnosis of Digestive Diseases
School of Medical Sciences, State University of Campinas
Campinas, São Paulo, Brazil

Section 1

# General Comments on H. pylori Infection and Extradigestive Diseases

Chapter 1

# Extra-digestive Manifestations of *Helicobacter pylori* Infection – An Overview

Sue K. Park

Additional information is available at the end of the chapter

http://dx.doi.org/10.5772/63226

**Abstract**

*Helicobacter pylori* (*H. pylori*) is well known as a group I human gastric cancer carcinogen by the International Agency for Research on Cancer. Although an exact causal relationship is unclear, *H. pylori* is expected to have been associated with non-digestive abnormal condition and/or diseases, such as metabolic syndrome, atherosclerosis and cardiovascular diseases, which have substantially lots of prior studies; adaptive immune response – related disorders, such as autoimmune thyroid diseases (ATDs), urticaria, atopy and asthma; and the other extra-digestive diseases, such as chronic obstructive pulmonary disease (COPD), migraine, anemia and hyperemesis gravidarum. This chapter overviews several groups of extra-digestive diseases by *H. pylori* infection and discusses the role of *H. pylori* in relation to the diseases in the viewpoint of causality.

**Keywords:** *Helicobacter pylori*, non- digestive diseases, overview, causality, relationship

## 1. Introduction

*Helicobacter pylori* (*H. pylori*), gram- negative spiral or curved bacillus, was discovered in 1982 by two pathologists, Barry Marshall and Robin Warren, the 1982 Nobel Prize awardees. Almost all patients had active chronic gastritis or gastroduodenal ulcer and thus the bacteria got attention as an important etiological factor of these diseases. Ironically, back to the past, Freedburg and Barron had first found the spiral organisms among gastrectomy patients in 1940, but the bacteria were forgotten for a long time due to failure to replication in other studies.

*H. pylori* is an established cause of chronic active or superficial gastritis, gastroduodenal ulcer disease, gastric adenocarcinoma and the mucosa-associated lymphoid tissue (MALT) lymphoma. The International Agency for Research on Cancer (IARC), a suborganization of the World Health Organization (WHO), classified the *H. pylori* as a group I human gastric cancer carcinogen (the meaning of definite carcinogen) in 1994. *H. pylori* chronic infection to gastric tissue results in carcinogenic environment or causes chronic inflammation, which leads to gastric carcinogenesis. Chronic *H. pylori* infection also induces gastric lymphoid follicles and trigger MALT lymphomagenesis of lymphoid expansion, which leads to MALT lymphoma.

Although only a few people (1–3%) with *H. pylori* chronic infection develop gastric cancer, *H. pylori* explains a 60–90% of gastric cancer in studies of population attributable fraction (PAF) estimation.

Prior studies showed that *H. pylori* is also expected to be associated with extra-digestive diseases. The first group of diseases is abnormal metabolic profiles such as insulin resistance, diabetes, hypertension, obesity and dyslipidemia, which are the components of metabolic syndrome. Consequently, the abnormal profiles are complexly influenced to increase the risk for cardiovascular diseases by atherosclerosis and vascular dysfunction. The second group of diseases is adaptive immune response–related disorders, such as autoimmune diseases including autoimmune thyroid diseases (ATDs), atopic disease, urticaria and asthma. The other group is on elusive knowledge, such as COPD, glaucoma, migraine, anemia and hyperemesis gravidarum.

The suggested mechanism, despite of inconclusive causal relationship, is as follows: Chronic *H. pylori* infection induces chronic inflammation, a complex biological response of the tissues to *H. pylori*. Inflammatory factors including cytokines interleukin (IL) and tumor necrosis factor (TNF), especially induced from chronic, low-grade inflammation, on the infection-inflammation pathway are common in pathogenesis of gastritis, atherosclerosis, metabolic syndrome, obesity and diabetes. These inflammatory factors produced in the inflamed gastric mucosa are continually secreted into the circulation, and they can affect metabolic profiles.[1] Therefore, chronic, low-grade inflammation by chronic *H. pylori* infection may induce extra-gastric diseases due to the effect of *H. pylori*–induced cytokines.

*H. pylori* infection and its transmission were related to low socioeconomic status (SES) such as poor hygiene, water contamination, and non-healthy lifestyles such as poor diet, smoking and physical inactivity. Usually people who were tested with *H. pylori* infection are those in middle SES class and over, and therefore, non-gastric diseases are also diagnosed in this class. Poor hygiene hypothesis seems to be no more proper for these populations in the association of *H. pylori* infection with non-gastric diseases.

Therefore, this chapter introduces extradigestive diseases by *H. pylori* infection and discusses critical issues in the *H. pylori* role in extradigestive diseases in the viewpoint of causality of *H. pylori* infection for these diseases.

## 2. Dyslipidemia

Dyslipidemia, such as high total cholesterol and/or triglyceride concentration or low high-density lipoprotein (HDL) level, is a component for metabolic syndrome (MetS). Abnormal lipid profile in *H. pylori*–infected subjects has been reported in several studies. A review paper for dyslipidemia using 8 related articles[1] showed that *H. pylori* infection patients had higher levels of plasma total cholesterol, low-density lipoprotein (LDL)-cholesterol and/or triglyceride, but lower levels of high-density lipoprotein (HDL)-cholesterol relative to non-infected patients. These conditions were significantly replicated in 5,077 Japanese men only in a large population study for *H. pylori* eradication therapy, but failed to replicate it in women due to small number of woman patients.[1, 2] However, Satoh et al. showed significant associations between *H. pylori* infection and LDL or HDL levels only in male subjects and there was no significant association between *H. pylori* seropositivity and triglyceride concentration in the same study.[2] It is postulated that overexpression of various cytokines, such as IL-6 and TNF-$\alpha$ by *H. pylori* infection, may stimulate production of fatty acids by activating lipoprotein lipase in adipose tissue. Successful eradication treatment of *H. pylori* may induce an increase of HDL and decrease of LDL and triglycerides, but the alteration of blood lipid profiles before and after eradication therapy is not consistent in the total five observational studies and clinical trials.[1]

## 3. Hypertension

Hypertension is a component of MetS. Various cytokines induced by *H. pylori* infection in gastric mucosa may stimulate the hypothalamus and brain stem, which leads to sympathetic activation by secretion of cortisol and adrenaline. The subsequent pathway may induce the high blood pressure.[3] Although Harvey et al. reported the significantly positive association of *H. pylori* infection with hypertension in the community-based Bristol helicobacter project with the 10,537 subjects, the relationship is likely to be the result by residual confounding factors. Although a paper for African people showed decreased levels of blood pressure levels after three weeks of *H. pylori* eradication treatment,[4] it is likely to be not causally related because the study is not placebo controlled and remains misclassification bias because *H. pylori* test is not performed after treatment.

## 4. Insulin resistance and diabetes

Insulin resistance (IR) is one of important componnents on type 2 diabetes mellitus (DM) pathogenesis. In a systematic review published in 2011, a significantly high homeostatic model assessment-insulin resistance (HOMA-IR) score in *H. pylori*–infected population than non-infected population was reported in seven cross-sectional analyses.[5] In two non-randomized trials for *H. pylori* eradication therapy, a study showed a beneficial effect of *H. pylori* eradication therapy with decreased IR score in successfully eradicated patient group, but the other study failed to prove it. The potential mechanisms are suggested as follows: Lipopolysaccharides from *H. pylori* link to the activation of Toll-like receptors (TLRs), expressed mainly in macrophages and dendritic cells, which results in energy harvesting, fat accumulation and consequently IR.[6] And higher inflammatory cytokines can inhibit insulin action on its receptor through phosphorylation of serine residues on the insulin receptor and consequently induce insulin insensitivity and resistance.[5]

However, despite of statistical association between *H. pylori* infection and IR, there is continually arguing among investigators. The reasons are due to inconsistent result in comparison of IR status in pre– and post–*H. pylori* eradication therapy in a systematic review.[5] There were three non-randomized trials: two reported beneficial effects of *H. pylori* eradication therapy in decreasing IR score,[7] but the others [8] reported non-association and non-changes in the levels of IR in pre- and post-therapy regardless of eradication treatment.[5-7]

Three meta-analysis papers were reported up to date. In a meta-analysis using 41 diabetes and non-diabetes comparison studies in 2013, *H. pylori* infection was reported to be higher in patients with diabetes compared with non-diabetic patients,[9] and in the other meta-analysis using 13 case-control studies published in the same year, *H. pylori* infection was also associated with a 2-fold higher risk for diabetes among 13 case-control studies and at 1.6-fold higher risk for diabetic nephropathy among 6 case-control studies.[10] Both meta-analyses showed the action of *H. pylori* infection was stronger in type 2 diabetes than in type 1 diabetes.[9, 10]

The first prospective cohort study, published in 2012, of 782 diabetes-free subjects with 5-year follow-up presented that *H. pylori*–infected subjects had 2.7-fold higher risk for type 2 diabetes relative to non-infected people.[10, 11] However the other prospective cohort study, published in 2012, with 10-year follow-up did not show significant association between *H. pylori* infection and DM.[10–12] Moreover, meta-analysis of two cohort studies did not show any relationship.

The inconsistency across the studies is due to non-overcoming reverse causation and recall bias. The positive result in the first cohort study may be due to the finding secondary to the higher proportion of other risk factors of diabetes in *H. pylori*–infected group relative to non-infected group. Considering the results of the two cohort studies, it can be inferred that the significant effect of *H. pylori* infection on the development of diabetes may exist in only earlier life within 5-year follow-up and disappear or weaken due to risk factors of diabetes for long-term follow-up. Thus, the debate in causality for the association between *H. pylori* infection and diabetes has been still around.

## 5. Obesity

Although changes in ghrelin, a peptide hormone produced in the gastrointestinal tract, in relation to appetite or weight gain and in leptin, a hormone secreted from adipose tissue, in relation to inhibition of hunger and storage of triglycerides in adipocytes are suggested to be associated between obesity and *H. pylori* infection, there was inconsistent association across prior observational studies. Although the data regarding association between obesity and *H. pylori* infection are uncommon, most of the studies are cross-sectional design, non-overcoming reverse causation. The prior results are controversial across studies such as positive relationship (more obese in *H. pylori* infected people relative to non-infected people) and non-relationship.[1] Body mass index (BMI) after successful *H. pylori* eradication is expected to be decreased. However two non-randomized[13, 14] and a randomized placebo-controlled trial studies showed that BMI after successful *H. pylori* eradication was rather increased.[12]

## 6. Metabolic syndrome

The metabolic syndrome (MetS) is a group of five components: central obesity (waist circumference ≥102cm or 40 inches in male and ≥ 35 inches in female); high blood pressure (≥130/85 mmHg, and fasting plasma glucose ≥6.1 mmol/L); triglyceride dyslipidemia (triglyceride levels ≥1.7mmol/L); HDL-cholesterol dyslipidemia (high density lipoprotein-C (HDL-C) <40mg/dl in male and <50mg/dL in female); and hyperglycemia (fasting plasma glucose ≥6.1 mmol/L). By the standard of the US National Cholesterol Education Program Adult Treatment Panel III (NCEP III), MetS requires at least three of the five components. Many studies concerned the association between *H. pylori* infection and extradigestive manifestation. Relation of *H. pylori* infection with the MetS was evaluated in several studies.

Nabiour et al. first evaluated the association between *H. pylori* infection and MetS in 2006.[13] Compared with the group not infected by *H. pylori*, the group with *H. pylori* infection showed 1.5-fold significantly elevated risk for the MetS in both men and women. Association between *H. pylori* eradication treatment and remission of the MetS was evaluated to investigate the effect of *H. pylori* infection on the pathogenesis of the MetS. According to the study among Black people by Longo-Mbenza et al.,[4] three components such as plasma glucose, systolic and diastolic blood pressure and HDL-cholesterol levels were significantly improved compared with baseline values after three weeks of *H. pylori* eradication treatment. However, the two studies are cross-sectional small-numbered design; it is not obvious whether the observed difference is due to the anti-inflammatory or confounded effects by other risk factors than *H. pylori* eradication effects.[4] Also prior studies for the association of *H. pylori* infection for each MetS component failed to show its clear relationship. Therefore, further cohort studies with larger sample size need to be performed to confirm the relationship between MetS and its components and *H. pylori* infection, especially infection to highly virulent *H. pylori* such as CagA-strain.

## 7. Atherosclerosis and related diseases

Recent data have implicated *H. pylori* in atherosclerosis. Atherosclerosis, arteriosclerotic vascular disease, is a condition of artery wall thickness by complex pathogenesis of invasion and accumulation of white blood cells (WBCs) and proliferation of intimal smooth muscle cells by fatty fibrinogen plaque. It occurres due to chronic inflammation of WBCs and is promoted by residues of dead cells, including cholesterol and triglycerides. It can increase cardiovascular and cerebrovascular morbidity and mortality.

Biologically, *H. pylori* infection to gastric tissue can induce inflammatory cytokines, such as c-reactive protein (CRP), IL-series including 1, 6, 18, etc, and TNF-$\alpha$, which leads to systemic inflammation. *H. pylori* infection can modify asymmetric dimethylarginine (ADMA) and inhibit absorption of vitamin $B_{12}$ and folic acid in stomach, which also causes hyperhomocysteinemia.

Moreover, a virulent *H. pylori* strain, vacuolating cytotoxin A (VacA)-secreting *H. pylori*, infection can directly stimulate hyperhomocysteinemia. Cross-reaction between *H. pylori* antigens such as cytotoxin-associated gene A (CagA) and heat shock proteins (HSPs) produces autoimmune response by realizing it as a molecular mimicry of autoimmune antigen. Systemic inflammation by cytokine reaction, cytokines themselves as pro-atherogenic mediators, prohyperhomocysteinemia and autoimmune response complexly affect, thereby causing dysfunctional microvessels and inducing growth of vascular epithelial cells. *H. pylori* infection can also increase dyslipidemia, oxidative stress, and platelet aggregation. Subsequently these processes complexly induce and aggravate atherosclerosis.[14, 15] Additionally, pro-atherogenic cytokines activate hypothalamus and brain stem, which subsequently increase sympathetic hormones such as cortisol and adrenalin and result in hypertension, insulin resistance and dyslipidemia. These sequential pathological conditions finally lead to the cardiovascular diseases such as ischemic heart disease and ischemic stroke.[17, 18]

A prior case-control study of atherosclerosis measured by carotid intima-media thickness showed that *H. pylori*–infected people had higher carotid intima-media thickness than non-infected people and *H. pylori* infection increased the risk for atherosclerosis.[14] A prospective cohort study for 5-year follow-up showed the CagA-strain–infected group had much higher changes in intima-media thickness of common carotid arteries (IMT-CCA) and even developed new atherosclerotic lesions.[16] This study suggests that *H pylori* infection, in particular the more virulent *H. pylori* infection of CagA-strain, can be associated with atherosclerosis risk, perhaps due to an enhanced immune inflammatory response.

In contrast, the link between *H. pylori* infection and ischemic heart disease and stroke seems to be still left as unresolved issue due to divergent results. There are two meta-analyses for ischemic heart disease and two meta-analyses for coronary heart disease (CHD) events or death up to date. For ischemic heart disease, the meta-analyses of 10 case-control studies published in 2006 and of 26 case-control studies published in 2015 presented that *H. pylori* infection was associated with 1.87-fold and 2.1-fold higher risk for ischemic heart disease, respectively.[17, 18] Liu et al.'s summary risk was consistent, regardless of ethnicity and age (range 1.75–2.29).[18] For CHD, a meta-analysis of 15 case-control studies, published in 2008, presented that CagA had a 2.1-fold higher risk for CHD (Zhang et al.), and the other meta-analysis of 3 cohort studies, published in 2008, also presented a 1.26-fold higher risk for CHD (Pasceri et al., 2006). However, most recent meta-analysis, published in 2015, of 19 prospective cohort studies reported a debatable result: the significant effect was weaker (only 11% increase in the risk of CHD) and existed in only patients' early lives within follow-up of 5 years and the association was not seen at 10-year follow-up due to masking effect by CHD risk factors (Sun).

Meta-analyses for ischemic stroke, two published in 2008 and one in 2006, respectively, summarized results from case-control and cross-sectional studies and reported an increasing risk for ischemic stroke by *H. pylori* infection (Wang et al., 2008, a 1.6-fold higher risk by *H. pylori* infection including CagA; Pasceri et al., 2006, a 2.4-fold higher risk by CagA strain infection; Zhang et al., 2008, a 2.7-fold higher risk by CagA strain infection). However, a recent meta-analysis of six cohort studies and four nested case-control/case-cohort studies failed to prove the association (Yu), regardless of CagA virulence, study design, number of pathogens, and study quality (Yu). Case-control or cross-sectional designs have a higher possibility in overwhelming risk by their small size and consequently selection bias and insufficient adjustment for confounders. Therefore, the summary risk in meta-analysis of prior case-control and cross-sectional studies may be augmented relative to real risk value. Association between *H. pylori* infection and the risk of ischemic stroke up to date seems to be inconclusive.

## 8. Adaptive immune response relating disorders

Autoimmune disease develops when adaptive immune response induced by *H. pylori*–infected cells develops and autoantibodies are pronouncing against self-antigens, such as thyroid antigens,[19] circulating IgE or alpha-chain of the high-affinity IgE receptor.[20] Autoimmune diseases by *H. pylori* infection, autoimmune thyroid diseases (ATDs) and chronic urticaria (CU) have been reported. For ATDs, a meta-analysis of seven observational studies involving a total of 862 patients, published in 2013, indicated that *H. pylori* infection, especially CagA, was associated with 1.92-fold higher risk for total ATDs, and there is no heterogeneity and publication bias. In subgroup analysis, *H. pylori* infection was at 4.35-fold higher risk for Graves' disease, while Hashimoto's thyroiditis was not associated with *H. pylori* infection.[19]

For urticaria, a meta-analysis of nine case-control studies with high quality indicated that *H. pylori* infection was at 1.36-fold higher risk for CU (no heterogeneity and publication bias).[20] However, both meta-analyses fundamentally did not overcome the possibility of confounders and the problem of reverse causation and bias in meta-analysis using case-control studies, although the findings suggest *H. pylori* potentially plays a part in the development of ATDs and CU.[22, 23]

For atopy/allergic disease, a meta-analysis of 17 case-control studies performed in Western countries, published in 2014, showed a significant inverse association of *H. pylori* infection, perhaps by link of a better hygiene related to decrease of *H. pylori* infection and the large spreading of atopic diseases.[21] The mechanism of allergy is different from ATD. *H. pylori* infection may evoke immune tolerance, which is an overactive Th2 response by lack of the Th1 response, which facilitates persistent infection and inhibits allergic T-cell responses.[21] This mechanism is applied to asthma. A meta-analysis, published in 2012, of five case-control studies failed to show an association between *H. pylori* infection and asthma,[22] while the other meta-analysis, published in 2013, of 14 case-control and cross-sectional studies showed the opposite result, which is a significant reduced risk for asthma by *H. pylori* infection (OR=0.84), but had significant heterogeneity across studies.[23]

## 9. Other extra-digestive diseases

For COPD and CB, a meta-analysis, published in 2015, of 16 studies demonstrated that *H. pylori* infection had a 2.07-fold and 1.57-fold increased risk for Chronic obstructive pulmonary disease (COPD) and chronic bronchitis (CB) risk, respectively. CagA-strain *H. pylori* infection had much higher risk for COPD up to 3.46-fold. There are no heterogeneity and publication bias.[24] Although *H. pylori* infection on the etiology of CB and COPD remains controversial, two hypothetical mechanisms are suggested: 1) *H. pylori* infection may cause direct lung tissue damage, which leads to COPD and chronic bronchitis; 2) *H. pylori* infection triggers both diseases through sequential reaction of inflammatory cytokines.[24]

For migraine, a meta-analysis[25], published in 2014, of five cross-sectional studies showed that *H. pylori* infection had significantly 1.92-fold higher risk. However there are heterogeneity and publication bias across studies. Despite of its inconclusive result, the suggested mechanism is that *H. pylori* infection in stomach triggers inflammation, which stimulates the gastrointestinal neuroendocrine cells to secrete neuroendocrine peptides because migraine originates from the gastrointestinal organ. This sequential process may result in migraine by the brain-gut axis.[25]

For iron deficiency anemia (IDA), a meta-analysis,[26] published in 2010, of 15 case-control studies showed that *H. pylori* infection had significantly 2.22-fold higher risk. However, *H. pylori* eradication therapy in five RCTs was not efficient in improving hemoglobin and ferritin levels.[26] Both meta-analysis results had a publication bias and heterogeneity across the studies. The association is not causally related because IDA is specifically related to *H. pylori* infection and confounded by other risk factors.

For hyperemesis gravidarum (HG), a meta-analysis,[27] published in 2015, of 32 cross-sectional and case-control studies demonstrated a significantly 3.34-fold higher risk by *H. pylori* infection; however, there is heterogeneity across the studies. Hypothetical pathogenic mechanism is that *H. pylori* infection induces oxidative stress status by increasing reactive oxygen species (ROS) and decreasing plasma antioxidants, such as vitamin C and antioxidant enzymes, such as superoxide dismutase (SOD), catalase (CT) and glutathione peroxidase (GSH-Px).[27]

## 10. Summary and Conclusion

Most studies for extra-digestive diseases up to date are cross-sectional or case-control studies, with small sample size. There are several cohort studies, but the results are diverse. Cross-sectional or case-control designs are more susceptible to bias than cohort or clinical trial design. *H. pylori* infection was diagnosed by different methods up to date, which cause different *H. pylori* infection prevalence according to each assay method and affect heterogenous meta-analysis result across studies. Therefore, evidence as to what impact the *H. pylori* infection, especially highly virulent *H. pylori* infection such as CagA-strain infection, would have on the development of extra-digestive diseases concerned in lots of prior studies seems to be inconclusive. Large-scale, multicenter-based prospective cohort or clinical trial studies are still required to clarify the etiology between H. pylori and extra-digestive diseases because of the limited number of studies included in meta-analysis, their small sample sizes and inclusion of study design with low quality on causality reasoning evidence.

## Author details

Sue K. Park[1,2,3]

Address all correspondence to: suepark@snu.ac.kr

1 Department of Preventive Medicine, Seoul National University College of Medicine, South Korea

2 Department of Biomedical Science, Seoul National University Graduate School, South Korea

3 Cancer Research Institute, Seoul National University, South Korea

## References

[1] Buzas GM. Metabolic consequences of Helicobacter pylori infection and eradication. World journal of gastroenterology : WJG 2014;20(18):5226-34.

[2] Satoh H, Saijo Y, Yoshioka E, et al. Helicobacter Pylori infection is a significant risk for modified lipid profile in Japanese male subjects. J Atheroscler Thromb 2010;17(10):1041-8.

[3] Harvey R, Lane A, Murray L, et al. Effect of Helicobacter pylori infection on blood pressure: a community based cross sectional study. BMJ 2001;323(7307):264-5.

[4] Longo-Mbenza B, Nkondi Nsenga J, Vangu Ngoma D. Prevention of the metabolic syndrome insulin resistance and the atherosclerotic diseases in Africans infected by Helicobacter pylori infection and treated by antibiotics. Int J Cardiol 2007;121(3):229-38.

[5] Polyzos SA, Kountouras J, Zavos C, et al. The association between Helicobacter pylori infection and insulin resistance: a systematic review. Helicobacter 2011;16(2):79-88.

[6] Eshraghian A, Eshraghian H, Ranjbar Omrani G. Insulin resistance and metabolic syndrome: is Helicobacter pylori criminal? Minerva Gastroenterol Dietol 2011;57(4):379-85.

[7] Gen R, Demir M, Ataseven H. Effect of Helicobacter pylori eradication on insulin resistance, serum lipids and low-grade inflammation. South Med J 2010;103(3):190-6.

[8] Vafaeimanesh J, Rajabzadeh R, Ahmadi A, et al. Effect of Helicobacter pylori eradication on glycaemia control in patients with type 2 diabetes mellitus and comparison of two therapeutic regimens. Arab J Gastroenterol 2013;14(2):55-8.

[9] Zhou XY, Zhang CL, Wu JB, et al. Association between Helicobacter pylori infection and diabetes mellitus: A meta-analysis of observational studies. Diabetes Res Clin Pr 2013;99(2):200-08.

[10] Wang F, Liu J, Lv ZS. Association of Helicobacter pylori infection with diabetes mellitus and diabetic nephropathy: A meta-analysis of 39 studies involving more than 20,000 participants. Scand J Infect Dis 2013;45(12):930-38.

[11] Jeon CY, Haan MN, Cheng C, et al. Helicobacter pylori Infection Is Associated With an Increased Rate of Diabetes. Diabetes Care 2012;35(3):520-25.

[12] Lane JA, Murray LJ, Harvey IM, et al. Randomised clinical trial: Helicobacter pylori eradication is associated with a significantly increased body mass index in a placebo-controlled study. Aliment Pharmacol Ther 2011;33(8):922-9.

[13] Nabipour I, Vahdat K, Jafari SM, et al. The association of metabolic syndrome and Chlamydia pneumoniae, Helicobacter pylori, cytomegalovirus, and herpes simplex virus type 1: the Persian Gulf Healthy Heart Study. Cardiovasc Diabetol 2006;5:25.

[14] He C, Yang Z, Lu NH. Helicobacter pylori-an infectious risk factor for atherosclerosis? J Atheroscler Thromb 2014;21(12):1229-42.

[15] Karbasi-Afshar R, Khedmat H, Izadi M. Helicobacter pylori Infection and atherosclerosis: a systematic review. Acta Med Iran 2015;53(2):78-88.

[16] Mayr M, Kiechl S, Mendall MA, et al. Increased risk of atherosclerosis is confined to CagA-positive Helicobacter pylori strains: prospective results from the Bruneck study. Stroke; a journal of cerebral circulation 2003;34(3):610-5.

[17] Pasceri V, Patti G, Cammarota G, et al. Virulent strains of Helicobacter pylori and vascular diseases: A meta-analysis. American heart journal 2006;151(6):1215-22.

[18] Liu J, Wang F, Shi S. Helicobacter pylori Infection Increase the Risk of Myocardial Infarction: A Meta-Analysis of 26 Studies Involving more than 20,000 Participants. Helicobacter 2015;20(3):176-83.

[19] Shi WJ, Liu W, Zhou XY, et al. Associations of Helicobacter pylori infection and cytotoxin-associated gene A status with autoimmune thyroid diseases: a meta-analysis. Thyroid : official journal of the American Thyroid Association 2013;23(10):1294-300.

[20] Gu H, Li L, Gu M, et al. Association between Helicobacter pylori Infection and Chronic Urticaria: A Meta-Analysis. Gastroenterol Res Pract 2015;2015:486974.

[21] Lionetti E, Leonardi S, Lanzafame A, et al. Helicobacter pylori infection and atopic diseases: is there a relationship? A systematic review and meta-analysis. World journal of gastroenterology : WJG 2014;20(46):17635-47.

[22] Wang Y, Bi Y, Zhang L, et al. Is Helicobacter pylori infection associated with asthma risk? A meta-analysis based on 770 cases and 785 controls. Int J Med Sci 2012;9(7):603-10.

[23] Zhou XY, Wu JB, Zhang GX. Association between Helicobacter pylori and asthma: a meta-analysis. Eur J Gastroen Hepat 2013;25(4):460-68.

[24] Wang F, Liu J, Zhang Y, et al. Association of Helicobacter pylori infection with chronic obstructive pulmonary disease and chronic bronchitis: a meta-analysis of 16 studies. Infect Dis (Lond) 2015;47(9):597-603.

[25] Su J, Zhou XY, Zhang GX. Association between Helicobacter pylori infection and migraine: a meta-analysis. World journal of gastroenterology : WJG 2014;20(40): 14965-72.

[26] Qu XH, Huang XL, Xiong P, et al. Does Helicobacter pylori infection play a role in iron deficiency anemia? A meta-analysis. World journal of gastroenterology : WJG 2010;16(7):886-96.

[27] Li L, Li L, Zhou X, et al. Helicobacter pylori Infection Is Associated with an Increased Risk of Hyperemesis Gravidarum: A Meta-Analysis. Gastroenterol Res Pract 2015;2015:278905.

Section 2

# Helicobacter pylori Infection and Oral Cavity

Chapter 2

# *Helicobacter pylori* Infection and Halitosis – Evidence, Hypothesis, and Korean Red Ginseng to Mitigate Its Effect

Kyu Hyun Han, Jong-Min Park, Young-Min Han, Joo Young Cho, Weon Jin Ko and Ki Baik Hahm

Additional information is available at the end of the chapter

http://dx.doi.org/10.5772/63091

## Abstract

Halitosis is a common and ignored condition, but in some, it is a disease-associated health problem, suggestive of overt disease conditions and hasaffected about 25–30% of world's population, bothering nonmedical social disturbance in many people. Although two kinds, pseudohalitosis and halitophobia, are also concerned, genuine halitosis originated from the oral cavity, such as gingivitis, caries, and poor oral hygiene, in 80% and the remaining 20% are extraoral sources of halitosis, which should not be ignored because of stigmata suggestive of overt tissue dysfunctions, for instance, poor nutrition and hygiene, alcohol abuse, smoking, and systemic illness such as chronic obstructive pulmonary disease, liver cirrhosis, diabetes mellitus, and chronic renal diseases. In this chapter, *Helicobacter pylori* (*H. pylori*)–associated halitosis as one of the extragastric manifestations is introduced. Since diagnostics of halitosis includes subjective methods (examiner's sense of smell) and objective methods (instrumental analysis), under the hypothesis of a possible relationship between *H. pylori* infection and objective halitosis, the real levels of volatile sulfur compounds (VSCs) in the breath showed significant correlation between VSC levels and the degree of *H. pylori*–associated erosive gastritis as well as gastric cancer. These findings are further validated through either measuring $H_2S$ level in gastric juices of *H. pylori*–infected gastritis or checking the expressions of cystathionine-γ-lyase (CSE) and cystathionine-β-synthase (CBS) responsible for $H_2S$ generation in biopsied stomach. The eradication of *H. pylori* significantly ameliorated halitosis, accompanied with significant reductions in gastric $H_2S$ levels ($p<0.01$). Korean red ginseng was very effective in either reducing *H. pylori*–associated H2S or alleviating halitosis in patients with *H. pylori*–associated chronic atrophic gastritis. Conclusively, *H. pylori* infection demonstrates to have an important relationship with the development of halitosis, and its eradication could possibly promote the improvement of this condition.

**Keywords:** Halitosis, *Helicobacter pylori*, volatile sulfur compounds, hydrogen sulfide, gastritis, gastroesophageal reflux disease

# 1. Introduction

## 1.1. Halitosis, pseudohalitosis, and halitophobia

Halitosis is a very common and unpleasant condition, affecting around 1/4–1/3 of the general population, which can be classified into the following three conditions, genuine halitosis, pseudohalitosis, and halitophobia based on their pathogenesis [1, 2]; genuine halitosis is usually related to an organic pathology, such as periodontitis, gingivitis, gastritis, and other systemic illness, and malodor molecules such as volatile sulfur compounds (VSCs) that arise usually from bacterial interactions generate the basis of oral malodor, such as hydrogen sulfide ($H_2S$), methyl mercaptan ($CH_3SH$), and dimethyl sulfide [$(CH_3)_2S$]. In addition, sulfur compounds, short-chain fatty acids, such as butyric acid ($CH_3CH_2CH_2COOH$), propionic acid ($CH_3CH_2COOH$), and valeric acid ($C_5H_{10}O_2$), diamines, including cadaverine [$NH_2(CH_2)_5HN_2$] and putrescine [$NH_2(CH_2)_4HN_2$], 1-proxy-2-propanol, phenyl compounds, such as indole, skatole, phyridiene, alkalines, ketones, and nitrogen-containing compounds, such as urea [$(NH_2)_2CO_2$] and ammonia ($NH_3$), may contribute to malodor of halitosis [3, 4]. When the concentration of these molecules in halitotic breath exceeds a threshold detected by objective methods, genuine halitosis can be diagnosed. Furthermore, pathologies of the tongue, poor oral hygiene, deep caries, and postnasal drainage are primarily associated with halitosis, in which condition, species such as *Peptostreptococcus anaerobius, Bacteriodes* spp., *Centipedia peritontii, Eubacterium* spp., *Topbium parvulum, Camplyobacter rectus, Eikenella corrodens, Eubacterium sulci, Fusobacterium nucleatum* or *periodonticum, Porphyromonas endodontalis* or *gingivalis, Solobacterium moorei, Bacteriodes forsythus, Treponema denticola,* and *Streptococcus salivariou* are well-known bacterial strains responsible for halitosis [5, 6]. Next, pseudohalitosis can be described as a situation where obvious malodor is not perceived by others, but only perceived by the patient, that is, patients who consider to have bad breath, but who does never been acknowledged by others, the patients with pseudo-halitosis often coinciding with depression and anxiety [7]. Finally, halitophobia is a situation when a patient complains about halitosis after the treatment of either genuine halitosis or pseudo-halitosis, even though no objective clues were documented. Therefore, patients with halitophobia are usually accompanied with vague psychiatric disturbance [2]. Although 0.5–1% of the adult population is affected with halitophobia during their social life, most patients with halitophobia frequently hop and hop from clinic/specialist to clinic/specialist in order to find an argument for their self-esteemed problem [8].

Halitosis relevant with practical clinical problems can be classified into the following two clinical situations according to origin, one is oral halitosis, around 90% in all, and the other is extraoral halitosis, remaining 10% among whole halitosis [9]. Since VSCs are responsible for halitosis irrespective of origin, in case of extraoral halitosis, VSCs generally generated from the body, travel to the lung through the vascular system, and pull out through breath from the alveoli. As another systemic diseases causing extraoral halitosis, liver disease, such as cirrhosis, hepatoma, and hepatic failure, uremia from end-stage renal disease, and metabolic disorder, such as diabetic ketoacidosis and other kinds of metabolic disorders had been reported. Also, excess food intake (food factors) like garlic or onion can be common etiology for halitosis [10, 11]. Among these system diseases, it must be kept in mind that halitosis can be a clue symptom suggestive of serious cancers, especially gastric, liver, and pancreatic cancer. Furthermore, halitosis can be one of the prominent extragastric manifestations suggestive of *Helicobacter pylori* (*H. pylori*)–associated ulcer or cancer because of the evidence showing correlation between VSCs levels and these gastric lesions [12, 13], about which detailed description will be followed. As nonoral cause of halitosis, sinusitis, tonsillitis, bronchiectasis, subphrenic abscess, esophageal diverticulum, pyloric stenosis, gastroesophageal reflux disease (GERD), and hepatitis are very common diseases relevant to halitosis encountered in clinic.

## 2. Halitosis provoked by gastrointestinal (GI) diseases

Apart from oral cavity, the GI tract diseases caused halitosis as presenting symptoms, though physician and patients still abusively believe that halitosis originates from the oral cavity or stomach. For instance, almost all patients suffering from some erosive changes in esophago-gastric organ, halitosis might be very common and earliest manifestation. In our earlier investigation [15], almost all patients with GERD or some degree of erosive gastritis, real levels of VSCs were significantly increased. Other examples of clinical diseases, such as pyloric stenosis, duodenal obstruction, aorto-enteric anastomosis, pharyngeal pouches, Zenker's diverticulum, and hiatal hernia, usually led to halitosis as usual clinical manifestations. Especially, GERD, achalasia, or other malabsorption syndromes may cause halitosis accompanied with other symptoms of retching and flatulence. In cases of intestinal obstruction, halitosis may be detectable because the first sign noticed to either patient's relatives or physician. Halitosis is usually noted after consuming dietary products, such as garlic, onions, and some spiced foods cause transient unpleasant odor or halitosis [14]. Yoo *et al.* [15] found that erosive changes in the esophago–gastro–duodenal mucosa were significantly correlated with increased levels of VSCs, suggesting that halitosis could be a symptom suggestive of the erosive diseases of the upper gut mucosa. In detail, as shown in Figure 1, erosive changes in the esophageal mucosa, erosive type GERD, were strongly associated with VSC levels, ascertaining the hypothesis that halitosis can be a potential biomarker for the discrimination between erosive GERD and nonerosive GERD, assuring the presence of erosive change in the lower EG junction [16]. In summary, GI pathology was very common in patients with halitosis as extraoral origin [17], approximately 50–60% among all gastroenterology patients. Conclusively, halitosis symptom, usually ignored as insignificant, should be investigated to search for etiology even in nondental area. Accompanied with halitosis, there has been a report [18] describing that *H. pylori* colonization of tongue mucosa increased incidence of atrophic glossitis and burning mouth syndrome, especially accompanied with halitosis.

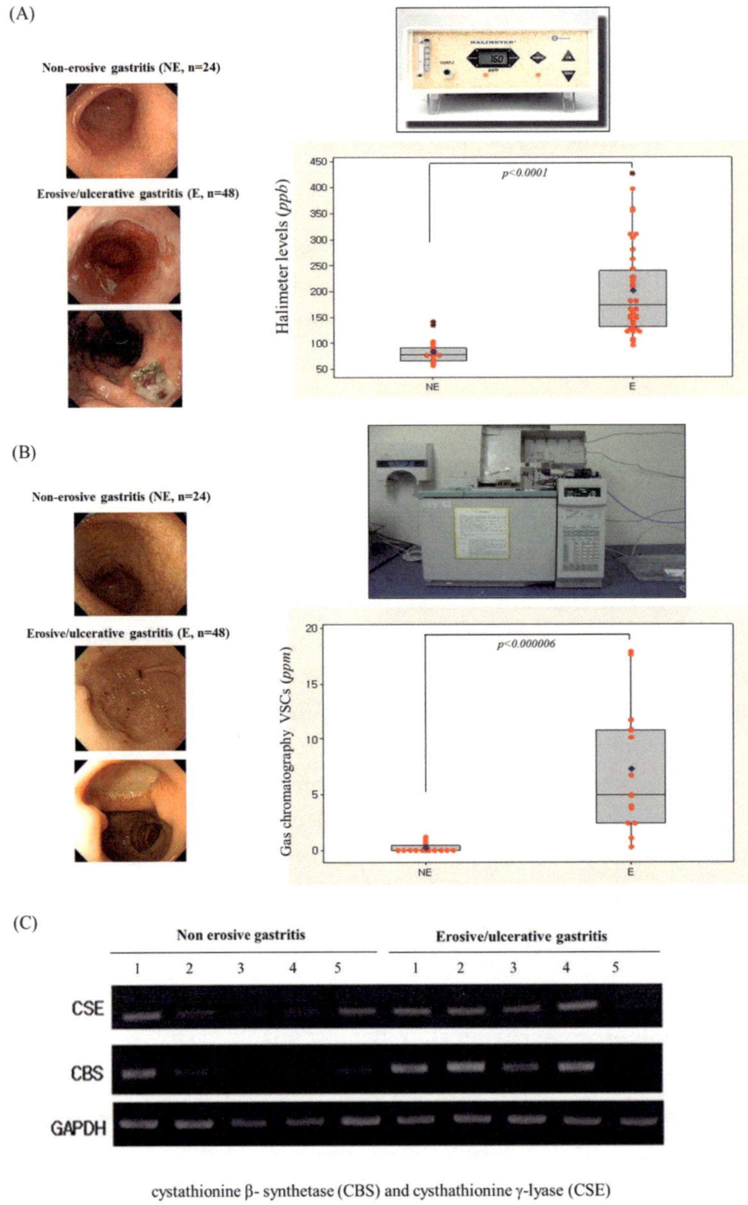


**Figure 1.** Correlation between EG lesion and halitosis. (A) Halitosis measurement with Halimeter in 72 patients with halitosis. Significant differences in Halimeter ppb were noted between patients with superficial gastritis and patients with erosive/ulcerative lesion (*p<0.0001*) (B) halitosis measurement with gas chromatography (GC) in same 72 patients with halitosis. Significant differences in VSCs ppm were noted between patients with superficial gastritis and patients with erosive/ulcerative lesion (*p<0.000006*). (C) The expressions of CSE and CBA according to EG mucosal changes. The mean expressions of CBS or CSE were significantly increasingly noted in patients with erosive changes. All of these results consistently suggested "halitosis" as possible biomarker predicting the presence of mucosal destruction and resulting putrefactive process in stomach.

## 3. Hydrogen sulfide ($H_2S$) biogas: Good, bad, ugly in its biology, and halitosis

Although biologic gas such as $H_2S$ as principal gas molecule is responsible for causing halitosis, there are contradictory biological implications of three major biogas, nitric oxide (NO), $H_2S$, and carbon monoxide (CO), in anti-inflammatory substances, promoting resolution of inflammatory processes, imposing several situations, including ischemic-reperfusion injury, cardioprotection, sepsis, hemostasis, fibrosis, pancreatitis, separately, but sometimes interacting each other [19, 20]. Interestingly, $H_2S$ stands for dual functions, inflammatory mediator or anti-inflammatory mediator [21], gaseous intracellular transducer implicated in either abnormal pathology or normal physiology [22], positioning homeostasis as friend or foe [23]. $H_2S$ and their responsible enzymes, cystathionine-β-synthase (CBS) and cystathionine-γ-lyase (CSE), played good or bad, but ugly biological implications dependent on cellular context and disease conditions.

Though many new technologies to detect endogenous $H_2S$ production and to develop novel $H_2S$-delivery compounds have been invented [24], simple gas with complex biology of good, bad, and ugly aspect, in this chapter, the way to detect VSCs, the implication of $H_2S$ among VSCs, and their regulations will be introduced. The Halimeter (Interscan corporation, Chatsworth, CA, Figure 1A) and OralChroma (Abimedical corporation, Kanagawa, Japan) are electronic devices available to detect some of the VSCs in expired air easily in clinic. These two devices are a portable gas chromatograph featuring easy to handle, lower cost, higher performance, time saving, fast results, very accurate, and reproducible even compared with conventional gas chromatographs. However, the limitation is that they limitedly target three gases: $H_2S$, $CH_3SH$, and $(CH_3)_2S$. With the Halimeter measurement, the total amount of VSCs in *parts per billion* (ppb) in breathing air is shown. In normal situations, this value is less than 100 ppb. When 300–400 ppb are detected in the mouth air, objective halitosis can be confirmed, of course, the changes of ppb level can be traced after some interventions to mitigate halitosis [25]. Though they are rather inexpensive and can be controlled by untrained staff, the limited diversity in the explored gasses and inconvenienceby examiner's cooperation should be further improved. On the other hand, the OralChroma may produce a more comprehensive assessment of VSCs production by oral microflora compared to Halimeter [26]. Of course, gas chromatography (GC) analysis can be performed on diverse sources, such as saliva, tongue debris, aspirated gastric juices, and even biopsied tissues, in addition to breath and almost all different air components can be detected, golden standard for halitosis, but not easy to measure and expensive [27]. In expired air, almost 500 different substances can be measured with GC (Figure 1B). Although GC has been used since the late 1960s, GC is still in an experimental stage, infrequent use for clinic [28]. Though GC has several advantages, such as an analysis of almost all components, high sensitivity, specificity, and noninvasive, it is very expensive, hard to handle because a well-trained staff is mandatory and not portably used [29]. Besides of these measurements, the scientific and practical value of additional or alternative measurement methods, such as benzoyl-DL-arginine-naphthylamide (BANA) test, chemical sensors, salivary incubation test, quantifying galactosidase activity, ammonia monitoring, Ninhydrin method, and PCR, has been applied in clinic.

### 3.1. $H_2S$ as dual-edged sword, is it neurotransmitter or inflammatory mediator?

$H_2S$ is a well-known toxic gas that is synthesized from the amino acids, cysteine and homocysteine, by two enzymes, CBS and CSE [30, Figure 1C]. Like other biogas, CO or NO, $H_2S$ is a signaling molecule implicated in either physiological actions of the cardiovascular or digestive system or pathophysiological actions in homeostasis, proliferation, and apoptosis of vascular smooth muscle cells, insulin release, nociceptive effects, cytoprotection, but contradictory action of inflammatory mediators, for instance, pancreatitis, chronic obstructive pulmonary disease, joint inflammation, sepsis, and *H. pylori*–associated gastritis in gastroenterology [23, 31–33]. In detail, in pancreatitis, especially in a form of severe acute pancreatitis (SAP), the fact that treatment with DL-propargylglycine (PAG) induced pancreatic acinar cell apoptosis and decreased the pathological scores as well as inflammatory parameters, whereas administration of NaHS significantly aggravated SAP suggested the implication of $H_2S$ in pancreatitis [34]. For instance, Bhatia M *et al.* [35] published that proinflammatory role of $H_2S$ regulated the severity of pancreatitis and even associated lung injury. On the other hand, in endotoxemia or sepsis model, $H_2S$ contributed to recovery or rescuing actions [36–38].

## 4. Halitosis as one of extragastric manifestations of *H. pylori* infection (Figure 3)

*H. pylori* was shown to produce $H_2S$ and $CH_3SH$, major oral malodor, inducing VSCs, suggesting that *H. pylori* can contribute to the development of halitosis relevant with tissue destruction in the GI tract [12]. The findings that as *H. pylori*–associated chronic gastritis worsened, it caused significant increase in levels of VSCs, but significant improvement of halitosis after eradication signified that halitosis can be overtly correlated with extra-gastric symptoms of *H. pylori* infection. Taken together with the additional fact that *H. pylori* infection was responsible for diverse oral pathologies [39], there are two liaisons between *H. pylori* infection and halitosis, one is that *H. pylori* can provoke halitosis through oral cavity infection [40] and the other is that gastric pathologies caused by chronic *H. pylori* infection are responsible for halitosis as extragastric manifestation [41]. According to literature search, there were 48 articles reporting the association between saliva/plaque and *H. pylori* infection. As example showing association between *H. pylori* infection and various oral diseases, Tiomny *et al.* [42] reported that in Israel, when studied six patients with halitosis and five of whom were *H. pylori* positive, the symptoms of halitosis disappeared after successful eradication. Similar results were reported by Ierardi *et al.* [43] documented with real measurement of VSC in *H. pylori* infection. Serin *et al.* [44] administered triple eradication therapy to subjects with *H. pylori*–positive halitosis and found about two third of patients were free from halitosis, all of these studies consistently signified that halitosis is a frequent and treatable symptom in *H. pylori*–positive chronic gastritis and can be a valid indication for *H. pylori* eradication. Our group extended these investigations, in which any erosive or ulcerative lesions relevant with *H. pylori* infection provoked higher rate of halitosis and healing from erosive changes warranted improvement of halitosis in all subjects, in this study objective measurements as well as subjective changes of halitosis were done with real value of $H_2S$ measured by either gas chromatography or Halimeter. Recently, it was reported that *H. pylori* infection increased the risk of BHH (burning, halitosis, and lingual dorsum hyperplasia). *H. pylori* detection in the oral cavity by histopathologic diagnosis and molecular biology was confirmed in 87% patients with BHH, but only lesser than 2.6% in other kinds of oral diseases [39,45].

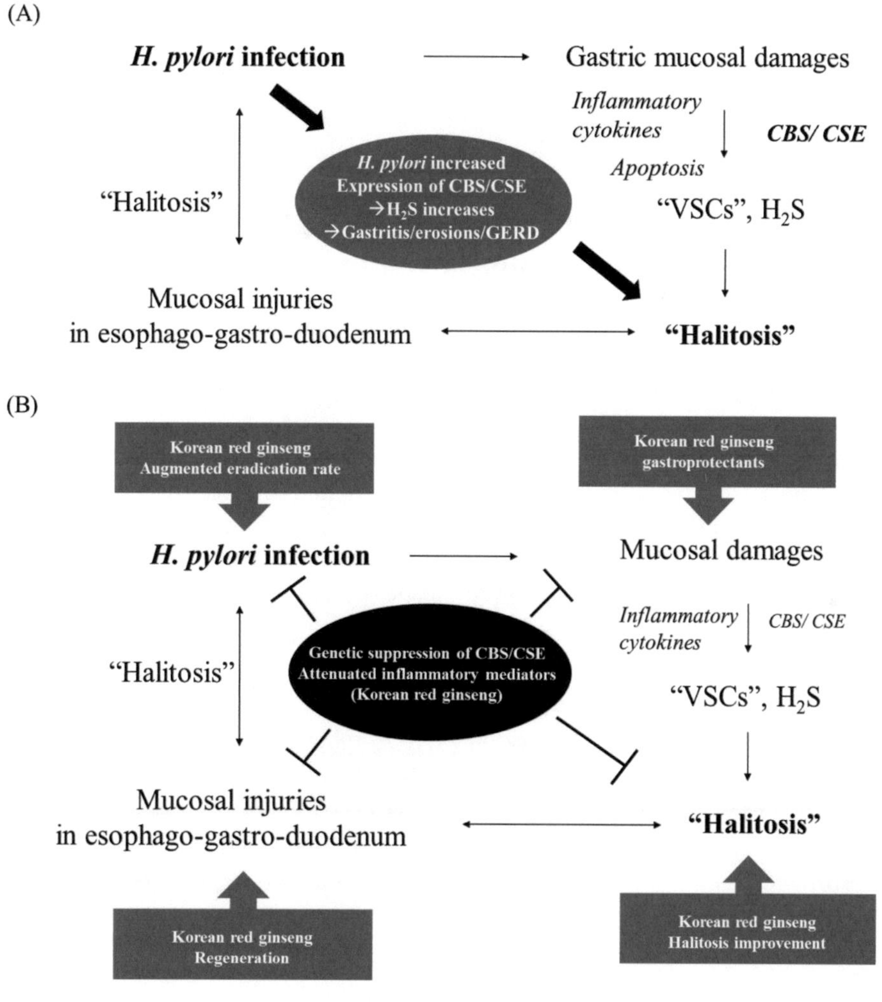


**Figure 2.** Halitosis as possible extragastric manifestation of *H. pylori* infection and relief with KRG. (A) *H. pylori* infection led to several pathogenic changes in gastric mucosa, oxidative stress, inflammatory mediators, apoptosis, and increasing expression of CBS and CSE, after which increased $H_2S$ seems to be responsible for inflammatory, ulcerative, and halitosis changes. (B) KRG was identified as natural product controlling CBS or CSE expressions followed with additional action mechanisms of augmenting eradication, lessening gastric inflammation, and ameliorating halitosis.

There were two translational studies confirming the association between *H. pylori* infection and halitosis through real measurements of VSCs in clinical setting: one was the study by Suzuki *et al.* [46] that used saliva from the 25 halitosis patients associated with *H. pylori* infection; the clinical symptoms associated with halitosis and periodontal symptoms were significantly greater in the *H. pylori*–positive subjects and the other from our author's group [15] shows that halitosis could be an effective biomarker in predicting *H. pylori*–associated erosive and inflammatory changes, of which were significantly correlated with halitosis improvement after eradication. Reports regarding the long-term outcome that eradication of *H. pylori* in patients with functional dyspepsia warranted sustained improvement of halitosis were available [47] and they strongly supported the existence of a close link between *H. pylori* infection and halitosis. Conclusively *H. pylori* eradication should be considered in patients with troublesome halitosis, bothering patients with limited social activities due to halitosis (Figure 2A).

## 5. Amelioration of troublesome halitosis through suppressing *H. pylori*–associated $H_2S$ with natural products

Lee *et al* [41] investigated 88 patients with functional dyspepsia presenting with halitosis, all of them showed very high levels of Halimeter >100 ppb, on whom tests were repeated after 10 weeks of Korean red ginseng (KRG) administration. As results, most patients with successful eradication of *H. pylori* benefited with subjective and objective improvement of halitosis. Before the current clinical trials, positive outcomes were anticipated in *in vitro* investigation that KRG extracts significantly decreased *H. pylori*- or NaHS-induced CSE expressions concomitant with attenuated levels of $H_2S$, IL-6, IL-8, as well as IL-1β mRNA. The findings that more than half of the cases (52.3–65.0%) became free of halitosis with KRG treatment alone, but it was the combination of a successful eradication regimen with KRG supplementation accompanied with *in vitro* proof showing KRG was very effective in suppressing the CSE/CBS gene led to the following conclusion: *H. pylori* infection might be closely responsible for halitosis and KRG supplementation was proven to be very effective in relieving halitosis in addition to being responsible for bacterial suppression (Figure 2B). In addition, generally good short-term results were reported with chlorhexidine. Triclosan seems less effective, essential oils and cetylpyridinium chloride are only effective up to 2 or 3 hours. Metal ions and oxidizing agents, such as hydrogen peroxide, chlorine dioxide, and iminium, are active in neutralizing volatile sulfur-containing compounds [48,49], but these are only for lessening halitosis not removing etiopathogenic background.

In conclusion, though the solution of halitosis problems must include the reduction of the intraoral bacterial load and/or the conversion of VSCs to nonvolatile substrates [50], targeting both etiologic organism removal and VSCs generating enzyme suppression seems to be very ideal modality of halitosis treatment (Figure 3), in which KRG seems to ideal product to deserve in clinic.

http://dx.doi.org/10.5772/63091

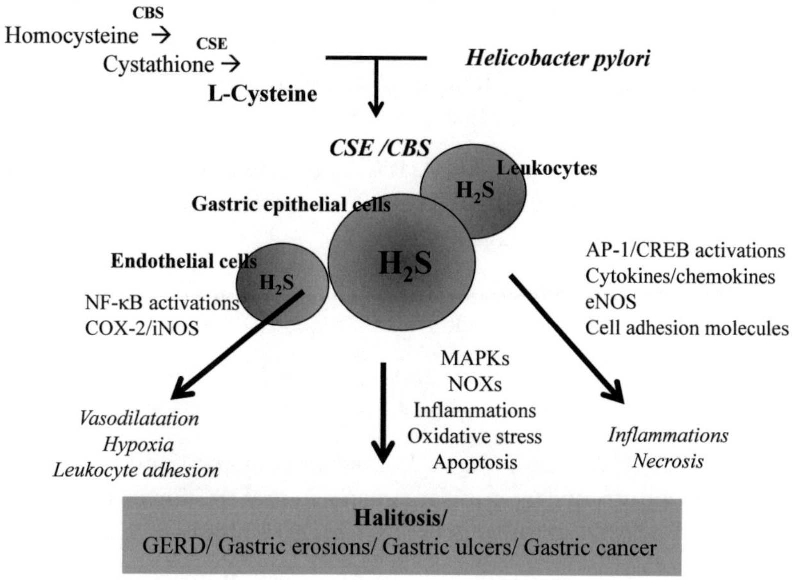


**Figure 3.** *H. pylorii* infection caused halitosis as well as overt clinical diseases relevant to $H_2S$ generation Dietary sources of L-cysteine and *H. pylori* infection provoked CBS/CSE activations, leading to increased $H_2S$ generation. Currently dual edged biological actions of $H^2S$ were reported; one was vasodilatation and antioxidative actions, and the other the aggravation of inflammations and hypoxic condition. In the stomach under *H. pylori* infection, $H_2S$-driven gastric surface destruction as well as gastritis finally rendered gastric diseases such as erosive gastritis or ulcerative lesions. Also halitosis was significantly manifested as extragastric symptoms associated with *H. pylori* infection due to significant associations and amelioration of halitosis after eradication.

## Acknowledgements

This study was supported by the grant from the Korea Society of Ginseng, funded from the Korea Ginseng Corporation (2012).

## Author details

Kyu Hyun Han[1], Jong-Min Park[2], Young-Min Han[2], Joo Young Cho[1], Weon Jin Ko[1] and Ki Baik Hahm[1,2*]

*Address all correspondence to: hahmkb@cha.ac.kr

1 Digestive Disease Center, CHA University Bundang Medical Center, Seongnam, Korea

2 CHA Cancer Prevention Research center, CHA Bio Complex, Seongnam, Korea

## References


[1] Gokdogan O, Catli T, Ileri F. Halitosis in otorhinolaryngology practice. Iranian Journal of Otorhinolaryngology. 2015;27(79):145–153.

[2] van den Broek AM, Feenstra L, de Baat C. A review of the current literature on aetiology and measurement methods of halitosis. Journal of Dentistry. 2007;35(8):627–635. DOI: 10.1016/j.jdent.2007.04.009

[3] Bollen CM, Beikler T. Halitosis: the multidisciplinary approach. International Journal of Oral Science. 2012;4(2):55–63. DOI: 10.1038/ijos.2012.39

[4] Hughes FJ, McNab R. Oral malodour--a review. Archives of Oral Biology. 2008;53(Suppl 1):S1–7. Epub 2008/06/14. DOI: 10.1016/s0003-9969(08)70002-5

[5] Kato H, Yoshida A, Awano S, Ansai T, Takehara T. Quantitative detection of volatile sulfur compound-producing microorganisms in oral specimens using real-time PCR. Oral Diseases. 2005;11(Suppl 1):67–71. DOI: 10.1111/j.1601-0825.2005.01096.x

[6] Donaldson AC, McKenzie D, Riggio MP, Hodge PJ, Rolph H, Flanagan A, et al. Microbiological culture analysis of the tongue anaerobic microflora in subjects with and without halitosis. Oral Diseases. 2005;11(Suppl 1):61–63. DOI: 10.1111/j.1601-0825.2005.01094.x

[7] Suzuki N, Yoneda M, Naito T, Iwamoto T, Hirofuji T. Relationship between halitosis and psychologic status. Oral Surgery, Oral Medicine, Oral Pathology, Oral Radiology, and Endodontics. 2008;106(4):542–547. DOI: 10.1016/j.tripleo.2008.03.009

[8] Nagel D, Lutz C, Filippi A. [Halitophobia--an under-recognized clinical picture]. Schweizer Monatsschrift fur Zahnmedizin = Revue mensuelle suisse d'odonto-stomatologie = Rivista mensile svizzera di odontologia e stomatologia/SSO. 2006;116(1):57–64.

[9] Tangerman A. Halitosis in medicine: a review. International Dental Journal. 2002;52 Suppl 3:201–206.

[10] Tangerman A, Winkel EG. Intra- and extra-oral halitosis: finding of a new form of extra-oral blood-borne halitosis caused by dimethyl sulphide. Journal of Clinical Periodontology. 2007;34(9):748–755. Epub 2007/08/25. DOI: 10.1111/j.1600-051X.2007.01116.x

[11] Lanzotti V. The analysis of onion and garlic. Journal of Chromatography A. 2006;1112(1–2):3–22. DOI: 10.1016/j.chroma.2005.12.016

[12] Lee H, Kho HS, Chung JW, Chung SC, Kim YK. Volatile sulfur compounds produced by *Helicobacter pylori*. Journal of Clinical Gastroenterology. 2006;40(5):421–426.

[13] Tangerman A, Winkel EG, de Laat L, van Oijen AH, de Boer WA. Halitosis and *Helicobacter pylori* infection. Journal of Breath Research. 2012;6(1):017102. DOI: 10.1088/1752-7155/6/1/017102

[14] Lu DP. Halitosis: an etiologic classification, a treatment approach, and prevention. Oral Surgery, Oral Medicine, and Oral Pathology. 1982;54(5):521–526.

[15] Yoo SH, Jung HS, Sohn WS, Kim BH, Ku BH, Kim YS, et al. Volatile sulfur compounds as a predictor for esophagogastroduodenal mucosal injury. Gut and Liver. 2008;2(2):113–118. DOI: 10.5009/gnl.2008.2.2.113

[16] Kim JG, Kim YJ, Yoo SH, Lee SJ, Chung JW, Kim MH, et al. Halimeter ppb levels as the predictor of erosive gastroesophageal reflux disease. Gut and Liver. 2010;4(3): 320–325. DOI: 10.5009/gnl.2010.4.3.320

[17] Kinberg S, Stein M, Zion N, Shaoul R. The gastrointestinal aspects of halitosis. Canadian Journal of Gastroenterology = Journal canadien de gastroenterologie. 2010;24(9): 552–556.

[18] Gall-Troselj K, Mravak-Stipetic M, Jurak I, Ragland WL, Pavelic J. *Helicobacter pylori* colonization of tongue mucosa--increased incidence in atrophic glossitis and burning mouth syndrome (BMS). Journal of Oral Pathology & Medicine. 2001;30(9):560–563.

[19] Magierowski M, Magierowska K, Kwiecien S, Brzozowski T. Gaseous mediators nitric oxide and hydrogen sulfide in the mechanism of gastrointestinal integrity, protection and ulcer healing. Molecules (Basel, Switzerland). 2015;20(5):9099–9123. DOI: 10.3390/molecules20059099

[20] Beltowski J. Hydrogen sulfide in pharmacology and medicine--An update. Pharmacological Reports. 2015;67(3):647–658. DOI: 10.1016/j.pharep.2015.01.005

[21] Wallace JL, Ianaro A, Flannigan KL, Cirino G. Gaseous mediators in resolution of inflammation. Seminars in Immunology. 2015;27(3):227–233. DOI: 10.1016/j.smim.2015.05.004

[22] Olas B. Hydrogen sulfide in signaling pathways. Clinica Chimica Acta; International Journal of Clinical Chemistry. 2015;439:212–218. DOI: 10.1016/j.cca.2014.10.037

[23] Olas B. Hydrogen sulfide in hemostasis: friend or foe? Chemico-Biological Interactions. 2014;217:49–56. DOI: 10.1016/j.cbi.2014.04.006

[24] Wang R. Physiological implications of hydrogen sulfide: a whiff exploration that blossomed. Physiological Reviews. 2012;92(2):791–896. DOI: 10.1152/physrev.00017.2011

[25] Rosenberg M, McCulloch CA. Measurement of oral malodor: current methods and future prospects. Journal of Periodontology. 1992;63(9):776–782. DOI: 10.1902/jop.1992.63.9.776

[26] Salako NO, Philip L. Comparison of the use of the Halimeter and the Oral Chroma in the assessment of the ability of common cultivable oral anaerobic bacteria to produce

malodorous volatile sulfur compounds from cysteine and methionine. Medical Principles and Practice: International Journal of the Kuwait University, Health Science Centre. 2011;20(1):75–79. DOI: 10.1159/000319760

[27] Tonzetich J. Direct gas chromatographic analysis of sulphur compounds in mouth air in man. Archives of Oral Biology. 1971;16(6):587–597.

[28] Larsson BT, Widmark G. A gas chromatographic method for analysis of volatiles in saliva samples. Acta Pharmaceutica Suecica. 1969;6(4):479–488.

[29] Tonzetich J, Coil JM, Ng W. Gas chromatographic method for trapping and detection of volatile organic compounds from human mouth air. The Journal of Clinical Dentistry. 1991;2(3):79–82.

[30] Kimura H. Hydrogen sulfide: its production and functions. Experimental Physiology. 2011;96(9):833–835. DOI: 10.1113/expphysiol.2011.057455

[31] Kimura H. Hydrogen sulfide: from brain to gut. Antioxidants & Redox Signaling. 2010;12(9):1111–1123. DOI: 10.1089/ars.2009.2919

[32] Kimura H. Hydrogen sulfide: its production, release and functions. Amino Acids. 2011;41(1):113–121. DOI: 10.1007/s00726-010-0510-x

[33] Bhatia M. Role of hydrogen sulfide in the pathology of inflammation. Scientifica. 2012;2012:159680. DOI: 10.6064/2012/159680

[34] Wang G, Han B, Zhou H, Wu L, Wang Y, Jia G, et al. Inhibition of hydrogen sulfide synthesis provides protection for severe acute pancreatitis rats via apoptosis pathway. Apoptosis : An International Journal on Programmed Cell Death. 2013;18(1):28–42. DOI:10.1007/s10495-012-0770-x

[35] Bhatia M, Wong FL, Fu D, Lau HY, Moochhala SM, Moore PK. Role of hydrogen sulfide in acute pancreatitis and associated lung injury. FASEB Journal: Official Publication of the Federation of American Societies for Experimental Biology. 2005;19(6): 623–625. DOI: 10.1096/fj.04-3023fje

[36] Bekpinar S, Develi-Is S, Unlucerci Y, Kusku-Kiraz Z, Uysal M, Gurdol F. Modulation of arginine and asymmetric dimethylarginine concentrations in liver and plasma by exogenous hydrogen sulfide in LPS-induced endotoxemia. Canadian Journal of Physiology and Pharmacology. 2013;91(12):1071-1075. DOI: 10.1139/cjpp-2013-0114

[37] Bekpinar S, Unlucerci Y, Uysal M, Gurdol F. Propargylglycine aggravates liver damage in LPS-treated rats: possible relation of nitrosative stress with the inhibition of H2S formation. Pharmacological Reports. 2014;66(5):897–901. DOI: 10.1016/j.pharep.2014.05.014

[38] Collin M, Anuar FB, Murch O, Bhatia M, Moore PK, Thiemermann C. Inhibition of endogenous hydrogen sulfide formation reduces the organ injury caused by endo-

toxemia. British Journal of Pharmacology. 2005;146(4):498–505. DOI: 10.1038/sj.bjp.0706367

[39] Adler I, Muino A, Aguas S, Harada L, Diaz M, Lence A, et al. *Helicobacter pylori* and oral pathology: relationship with the gastric infection. World Journal of Gastroenterology. 2014;20(29):9922–9235. DOI: 10.3748/wjg.v20.i29.9922

[40] Czesnikiewicz-Guzik M, Karczewska E, Bielanski W, Guzik TJ, Kapera P, Targosz A, et al. Association of the presence of *Helicobacter pylori* in the oral cavity and in the stomach. Journal of Physiology and Pharmacology : An Official Journal of the Polish Physiological Society. 2004;55 Suppl 2:105-115.

[41] Lee JS, Kwon KA, Jung HS, Kim JH, Hahm KB. Korea red ginseng on *Helicobacter pylori*-induced halitosis: newer therapeutic strategy and a plausible mechanism. Digestion. 2009;80(3):192—199. DOI: 10.1159/000229997

[42] Tiomny E, Arber N, Moshkowitz M, Peled Y, Gilat T. Halitosis and *Helicobacter pylori*. A possible link? Journal of Clinical Gastroenterology. 1992;15(3):236–237.

[43] Ierardi E, Amoruso A, La Notte T, Francavilla R, Castellaneta S, Marrazza E, et al. Halitosis and *Helicobacter pylori*: a possible relationship. Digestive Diseases and Sciences. 1998;43(12):2733–2737.

[44] Serin E, Gumurdulu Y, Kayaselcuk F, Ozer B, Yilmaz U, Boyacioglu S. Halitosis in patients with *Helicobacter pylori*-positive non-ulcer dyspepsia: an indication for eradication therapy? European Journal of Internal Medicine. 2003;14(1):45–48.

[45] Adler I, Denninghoff VC, Alvarez MI, Avagnina A, Yoshida R, Elsner B. *Helicobacter pylori* associated with glossitis and halitosis. Helicobacter. 2005;10(4):312–317. DOI: 10.1111/j.1523-5378.2005.00322.x

[46] Suzuki N, Yoneda M, Naito T, Iwamoto T, Masuo Y, Yamada K, et al. Detection of *Helicobacter pylori* DNA in the saliva of patients complaining of halitosis. Journal of Medical Microbiology. 2008;57(Pt 12):1553–1559. DOI: 10.1099/jmm.0.2008/003715-0

[47] Katsinelos P, Tziomalos K, Chatzimavroudis G, Vasiliadis T, Katsinelos T, Pilpilidis I, et al. Eradication therapy in *Helicobacter pylori*-positive patients with halitosis: long-term outcome. Medical Principles and Practice: International Journal of the Kuwait University, Health Science Centre. 2007;16(2):119–123. DOI: 10.1159/000098364

[48] Krespi YP, Shrime MG, Kacker A. The relationship between oral malodor and volatile sulfur compound-producing bacteria. Otolaryngology--head and neck surgery : Official Journal of American Academy of Otolaryngology-Head and Neck Surgery. 2006;135(5):671–676. DOI: 10.1016/j.otohns.2005.09.036

[49] van den Broek AM, Feenstra L, de Baat C. A review of the current literature on management of halitosis. Oral Diseases. 2008;14(1):30–39. DOI: 10.1111/j.1601-0825.2006.01350.x

[50] Cortelli JR, Barbosa MD, Westphal MA. Halitosis: a review of associated factors and therapeutic approach. Brazilian Oral Research. 2008;22 Suppl 1:44–54.

Section 3

# Hematological Diseases and H. pylori Infection

Chapter 3

# *Helicobacter pylori* and Hematologic Diseases

Germán Campuzano-Maya

Additional information is available at the end of the chapter

http://dx.doi.org/10.5772/62971

**Abstract**

*Helicobacter pylori* infection is the most common infection of the human species, with developing countries displaying a marked disadvantage in contrast to developing countries. While *H. pylori* infection is asymptomatic in most infected individuals, it is intimately related to malignant diseases of the stomach, such as gastric cancer and gastric MALT lymphoma, as well as benign diseases, for example chronic gastritis and duodenal and gastric peptic ulcers. Since the discovery that gastric mucosa could be colonized by bacteria, evidence of greater than 50 extragastric manifestations has been reported, linking *H. pylori* infection and the development of diseases associated with cardiology, dermatology, endocrinology, obstetrics and gynecology, hematology, pneumology, neurology, odontology, ophthalmology, otorhinolaryngology, and pediatrics. This chapter presents the extragastric manifestations of *H. pylori* infection expressed through hematologic diseases; particularly those included in the international consensus, and discusses guidelines for the management of *H. pylori* infection, such as iron deficiency, vitamin $B_{12}$ (cobalamin) deficiency, and immune thrombocytopenia. Other manifestations reviewed include immune neutropenia, antiphospholipid syndrome, and plasma cell dyscrasias, such us monoclonal gammopathy of undetermined significance, multiple myeloma, and Henoch–Schönlein purpura.

**Keywords:** *Helicobacter pylori*, iron deficiency, immune thrombocytopenia, mucosa-associated lymphoid tissue lymphoma, vitamin $B_{12}$ deficiency

## 1. Introduction

*Helicobacter pylori* infects greater than 50% of the world population's stomachs, therefore constituting the most common infection of the human species [1]. A marked disadvantage exists between developed countries, where the prevalence ranges between 30% and 50%, and developing countries, where the prevalence ranges between 80% and 90% [2]. Since the discovery in 1983 that the stomach could be colonized by bacteria [3], sufficient evidence has accumulated implicating *H. pylori* as a pathogen intimately related to benign stomach diseases, such us chronic gastritis and duodenal and gastric peptic ulcers [3], and malignant diseases, for example gastric cancer [4] and gastric MALT lymphoma [5]. Furthermore, during the last three decades following the discovery [3], approximately 50 extragastric diseases have been reported in medical specialties such as cardiology, dermatology, endocrinology, obstetrics and gynecology, pneumology, neurology, odontology, ophthalmology, otorhinolaryngology, pediatrics, and hematology [6-20], the last of which is the subject of this review.

From a practical standpoint, hematological associations with *H. pylori* infection can be arbitrarily divided into two groups: (1) hematological diseases with sufficient scientific evidence to be recognized by the consensus and guidelines for the management of *H. pylori* among the indications of study and eradication and (2) hematological diseases where there is suspicion, with greater or lesser scientific evidence, of an association with *H. pylori* infection. Table 1 presents the hematological diseases associated with or possibly associated with *H. pylori* infection.

| **Recognized manifestations** |
| --- |
| Iron deficiency |
| Vitamin $B_{12}$ deficiency |
| Immune thrombocytopenia |
| Gastric MALT lymphoma |
| **Unrecognized manifestations** |
| Autoimmune neutropenia |
| Antiphospholipid syndrome |
| Plasma cell dyscrasias |
| Henoch–Schönlein purpura |
| Other manifestations: acute leukemia, myelodysplastic syndrome, thrombocytosis |

**Table 1.** Hematologic manifestations of *H. pylori* infection

## 2. Hematological diseases recognized as related to *H. pylori*

Until September 2015, the scientific community has recognized three hematologic diseases as extragastric manifestations of *H. pylori* infection: iron deficiency [21-30], vitamin $B_{12}$ deficiency [27, 29], and immune thrombocytopenia (ITP) [21, 23-31]. These will be carefully analyzed in the following subsections. Gastric MALT lymphoma, although considered a disease in the oncohematologic field and is associated with *H. pylori* infection, is not presented in this review because it is recognized as gastric manifestation.

### 2.1. Iron deficiency

Iron deficiency, with or without anemia (*anemia sine anemia*), is a serious public health problem, which affects approximately 25% of the world's population (greater than two billion people), according to the World Health Organization (WHO). Importantly, it mainly affects disadvantaged populations, such as children and women of gestational age [32, 33]. Iron deficiency, with or without anemia, is associated with increased morbidity due to high susceptibility to infections, decreased labor productivity, delayed weight–height and cognitive development, and other conditions [34].

It is important to note that iron deficiency is a chronic process: an iron imbalance can take several years to become established and manifest clinically or through hemogram (blood cell count) parameters, such as morphological alterations of erythrocytes or anemia, according to the WHO criteria [32]. Three stages of iron deficiency are clearly established: prelatent (Stage 1), when serum ferritin is between 12 μg/L and 30 μg/L; latent (Stage 2), when serum ferritin is below 12 μg/L; and iron deficiency anemia (Stage 3), when anemia is observed in addition to diminished or depleted iron storage levels determined by serum ferritin [35].

### *2.1.1. H. pylori and iron deficiency*

In 1991, in Belgium, Blecker et al. described the first association between iron deficiency and *H. pylori* infection. The patient was a 15-year-old young with iron deficiency anemia (hemoglobin 8.5 g/dL) secondary to chronic active hemorrhagic gastritis, positive to *H. pylori*, without prior gastrointestinal manifestations, in whom after *H. pylori* eradication the hematologic parameters and ferrokinetics test returned to normal without requiring supplemental iron treatment [36]. Two years later, in France, Bruel et al. reported a second case of iron deficiency anemia (hemoglobin 5.6 g/dL), in an 11-year-old child, which manifested as an upper gastrointestinal hemorrhage with documented infection with *H. pylori*. The anemia was resolved after eradication of the infection, again without supplemental iron treatment [37]. In the same year, in Italy, Dufour et al. presented the case of a 7-year-old boy diagnosed with refractory iron deficiency anemia (hemoglobin 5.1 g/dL), who had been treated with oral iron, the presence of *H. pylori* was reported and was asymptomatic from the viewpoint of gastrointestinal manifestations. As in the preceding cases, the infection was eradicated without supplementary iron treatment and the hematologic parameters, including hemoglobin (13.0 g/dL), returned to normal after 6 months [38].

After these first reports, where iron deficiency disappeared after the eradication of *H. pylori* [36-38], new isolated cases were published in last century [39-43], which as the first series demonstrate the association of *H. pylori* with iron deficiency and iron deficiency anemia [40, 44, 45]. The first decade of the twenty-first century provided most of the studies that currently support the five meta-analyses associating *H. pylori* infection with iron deficiency and the resolution of disease following infection eradication [46-50] in children [51-60], in pubescent males and females [61, 62], in prepubertal girls [63], in adult men and women [40, 45, 64-75], in seniors [76], in pregnant women [63], and in non-pregnant women [77]. In addition, these studies have provided scientific support to the different consensus and guidelines for incorporating iron deficiency into the medical management of *H. pylori* infection as an extragastric manifestation and indication for eradication [21-30].

### *2.1.2. Pathophysiology of iron deficiency by H. pylori*

The pathophysiological mechanisms through which *H. pylori* is associated with the etiology of iron deficiency, with or without anemia, has not been fully elucidated, and more questions remain than answers. Possible explanations proposed to clarify the association between *H. pylori* and iron deficiency will be enunciated. However, it is not yet known why this association exists in some patients but not in others, where a different association is presented or the infection is asymptomatic, as happens in most cases [78].

In the past decade, *H. pylori* infection and iron deficiency have been linked through a recently discovered hormone called hepcidin [79]. Hepcidin is a hormone of hepatic origin that regulates iron absorption at the enterocyte level in the small intestine and the liberation of stored iron from the macrophages of reticuloendothelial system [80]. Hepcidin is elevated, as an acute phase reactant, in response to inflammation in the gastric mucosa. This in turn translates into a physiological iron deficiency, known clinically as anemia of chronic inflammation [81-85]. Preliminary studies show that serum hepcidina levels are elevated in patients infected with *H. pylori* [85-87] and return to normal after eradication of the infection [88], thereby permitting iron absorption in enterocytes and liberation from entrapment in the macrophage reticuloendothelial system.

Other possible causes of iron imbalance in patients infected with *H. pylori* can result from chronic gastritis, which occurs in all infected individuals [78]. This condition can generate bleeding when transforms into erosive gastritis [89], especially in patients with bleeding duodenal or gastric peptic ulcers [90, 91] and in patients who chronically consume non-steroidal anti-inflammatory drugs (NSAIDs), including aspirin, for the purpose of cardiopro-tection [92-95]. Other mechanisms invoked to explain iron deficiency in patients infected with *H. pylori* are related to changes in gastric physiology, particularly changes in gastric pH and the presence of achlorhydria, which significantly reduces the solubility and intestinal absorp-tion of inorganic iron [40].

Beyond the aforementioned evidence, certain highly virulent strains of *H. pylori*, such as those with cytotoxin-associated gene A (CagA) and vacuolating cytotoxin gene A (VacA), which act through molecular mimicry mechanisms, are more likely to develop or magnify iron deficiency in infected patients, compared with infected patients with strains not carrying these genes [71, 96-98]. This situation could explain, in part, the marked differences from one region to another and the large discrepancies observed in different studies.

### *2.1.3. Management of iron deficiency in the post-Helicobacter era*

Regarding to the management of iron deficiency in the post-*Helicobacter* era, it is important to clarify that *H. pylori* is not the only cause of iron deficiency, and its incorporation into the consensus and management guidelines of *H. pylori* as an indication to investigate and eradicate the infection is not a substitute for an adequate study of the most common causes of iron deficiency. These situations are particular to each region, according to prevalence of iron deficiency and *H. pylori* infection, which vary from place to place. Thanks to over 250 referenced studies in the literature aiming to clarify different aspects of the association between *H.*

*pylori* and the development of iron deficiency, five meta-analyses are now available that demonstrate the impact of infection on the development of iron deficiency and that infection eradication improves hematological parameters and ferrokinetics [46-50]. These analyses have enabled the scientific community, particularly the consensus and management guides, to incorporate iron deficiency of unexplained origin as an indication to evaluate and eradicate *H. pylori* infection, when present, in adults as well as children [21-30].

Before initiating treatment for a patient with iron deficiency, an assessment of the prevalence of *H. pylori* infection should be performed according to region. Generally, the prevalence is low in developed countries; these cases should proceed with conventional management of iron deficiency [32, 35]. In developing countries, the rate of *H. pylori* infection is high; in these cases or when the patient, despite living in a country where infection rates are low, comes from a country where the infection rates are high, it should proceed to determine the status of *H. pylori* through a non-invasive test, ideally the $^{13}C$-urea breath test [27]. If the patient is negative for *H. pylori*, it is necessary to investigate other causes of the iron deficiency and treat the patient conventionally [32, 35], whereas if the patient is positive for *H. pylori*, it is indispensable to eradicate the infection [27].

After 6–8 weeks of treatment, the infection eradication must be confirmed using a non-invasive test, ideally with $^{13}C$-urea breath test [27]. If eradication is not achieved, it is mandatory to establish a new therapy scheme until eradication is achieved. Once *H. pylori* eradication is achieved and an improvement in hematological parameters and ferrokinetics (complete or partial remission) is obtained, it is important to periodically evaluate the clinical hematological parameters and the indicators of iron levels. If there is no response, it must establish a conventional management of iron deficiency [32, 35].

Figure 1 shows a diagnostic and management algorithm of iron deficiency in the post-*Helicobacter* era, taking into account the prevalence of infection and *H. pylori* status.

### 2.2. Vitamin $B_{12}$ deficiency

Vitamin $B_{12}$, also known as cobalamin, is a coenzyme necessary for the metabolism of amino acids, such as methionine, threonine, and valine, and for DNA synthesis through the conversion of methyl-tetrahydrofolate to tetrahydrofolate [99]. Vitamin $B_{12}$ is synthesized in mammals, but for humans, their provision depends exclusively of diet intake of animal products [99].

Again, as with iron deficiency, it should be noted that vitamin $B_{12}$ deficiency is a chronic process, with very slow establishment. It may manifest clinically through neuropsychiatric symptoms or through hemogram parameters, such as morphological alterations of erythrocytes or anemia, according to the WHO criteria [32]. Four stages of vitamin $B_{12}$ deficiency are clearly established: Stage I, reduction of vitamin $B_{12}$ levels in blood; Stage II, low amount of vitamin $B_{12}$ cellular levels and metabolic disorders; Stage III, increase in homocysteine and methylmalonic acid levels and decrease in DNA synthesis with onset of neuropsychiatric symptoms; and Stage IV, macrocytic anemia [100].

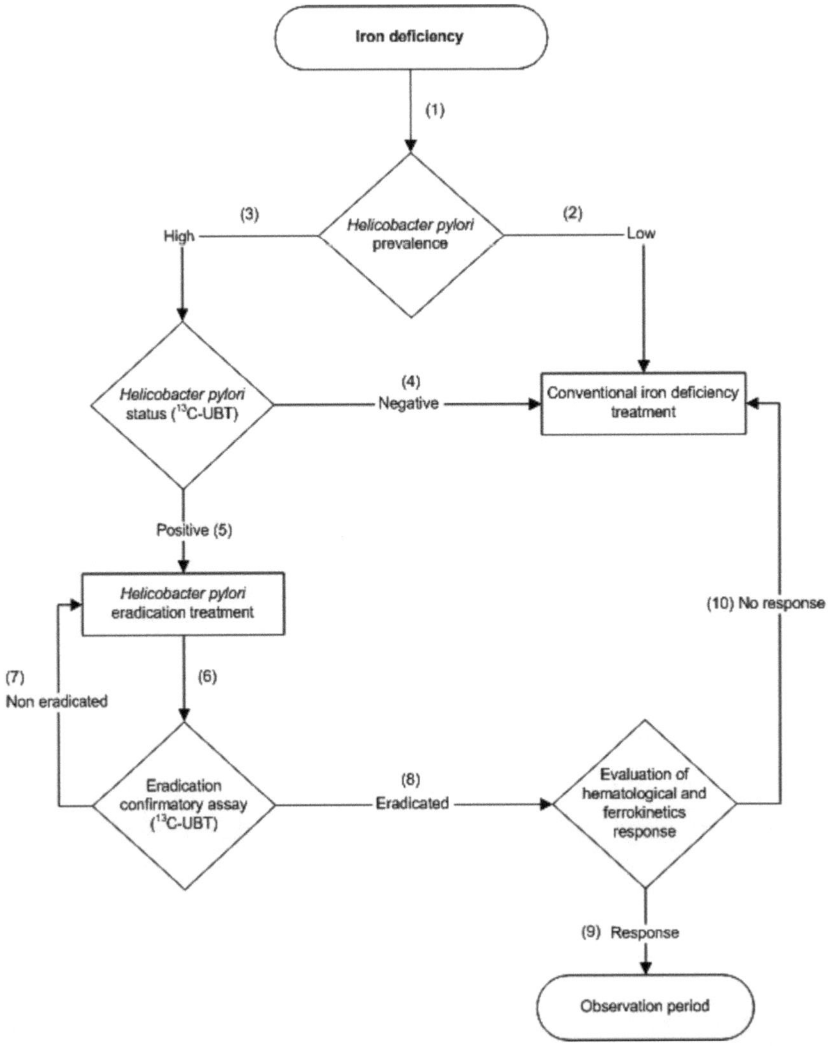


**Figure 1.** Algorithm for the study and management of iron deficiency, with or without anemia, in the post-*Helicobacter* era. (1) Before initiating treatment for a patient with iron deficiency, an assessment of the prevalence of *H. pylori* infection should be performed in each region. Generally, it is high in developing countries and low in developed countries [1]. (2) If the rates of *H. pylori* infection are low, proceed with a conventional management of iron deficiency [32, 35]. (3) If the rates of *H. pylori* infection are high or the patient, despite living in a country where infection rates are low, comes from a country where the infection rates are high, proceed to determine the status of *H. pylori* through a non-invasive test, ideally the $^{13}$C-urea breath test ($^{13}$C-BUT) [27]. (4) If the patient is negative for *H. pylori*, investigate other causes of the iron deficiency and treat conventionally [32, 35]. (5) If the patient is positive for *H. pylori*, proceed with eradication of the infection [27]. (6) Confirm infection eradication 6–8 weeks after the treatment using a non-invasive test, ideally with the $^{13}$C-urea breath test [27]. (7) If eradication is not achieved, establish a new scheme of eradication therapy until it is achieved. (8) Once *H. pylori* eradication is achieved, (9) if a response is obtained in the hematological parameters and ferrokinetics (complete or partial remission), periodically evaluate the clinical hematological parameters and indicators of iron. (10) If there is no response, proceed with a conventional management of iron deficiency [32, 35].

Vitamin $B_{12}$ deficiency is defined in terms of the serum values of vitamin $B_{12}$ and two components of its metabolic pathway, homocysteine and methylmalonic acid [101]. The diagnosis of vitamin $B_{12}$ deficiency is established in accordance with the following criteria: (1) serum vitamin $B_{12}$ < 150 pmol/L (< 200 pg/mL) with clinical manifestations and/or hematological alterations related to vitamin $B_{12}$ deficiency; (2) serum vitamin $B_{12}$ < 150 pmol/L, measured on two separate occasions; (3) serum vitamin $B_{12}$ < 150 pmol/L and serum homocysteine > 13 mmol/L or urinary methylmalonic acid > 0.4 mmol/L (in the absence of renal failure, folic acid deficiency, and vitamin $B_6$ deficiency); and (4) levels of serum holotranscobalamin < 35 pmol/L [102].

The prevalence of vitamin $B_{12}$ deficiency is highly variable and represents a serious public health problem, depending on the populations analyzed. Epidemiologic studies show that, in the general population of industrialized countries, vitamin $B_{12}$ deficiency has a prevalence of approximately 20%, with a range between 5% and 60%, depending on the definition of vitamin $B_{12}$ deficiency that is utilized [101, 102]. The prevalence of vitamin $B_{12}$ deficiency expressed as pernicious anemia is higher in Latin American countries than in the rest of the world; furthermore, in Latin America, the disease occurs in younger persons [103], while it is associated with advanced age in remaining countries [104].

In addition to its close association to the etiology of pernicious anemia [105] and subacute combined degeneration [106], vitamin $B_{12}$ deficiency is related, through homocysteine, with dissimilar diseases such as Alzheimer's disease [107, 108], dementia [109, 110], depression [111], stroke [112, 113], pulmonary embolism [114, 115], acute myocardial infarction, and coronary heart disease [116].

### 2.2.1. *H. pylori and vitamin $B_{12}$ deficiency*

The possibility that pernicious anemia, rather than vitamin $B_{12}$ deficiency, was associated with *H. pylori* was the first extragastric association postulated within the scientific community. This postulation was made by O'Connor et al. in 1984 [117], a year after Warren and Marshall inform the scientific community that the stomach could be colonized by bacteria [3]. Despite this premature interest, the association has been difficult to sustain and, rather, has been denied by many authors. Fong and colleagues performed what is considered the first well-founded study to clarify the probable link between *H. pylori* infection and pernicious anemia. In this study, the authors concluded that patients that suffer pernicious anemia are protected against *H. pylori* infection and that the bacteria not invade the inflamed mucosa by isolated processes [118]. These data were ratified in a Japanese study made by Saito et al. [119] and have been shared by other authors, however, with the wrong conclusion [120].

It is currently known that when vitamin $B_{12}$ deficiency becomes clinically relevant, the bacteria are no longer at the site of the lesion due to changes in the gastric mucosa that result in a hostile environmental niche. In cases of vitamin $B_{12}$ deficiency and pernicious anemia, *H. pylori* disappears as a result of changes mediated by the immunological response. These changes can be evidenced by the presence of antibodies against parietal cells and intrinsic factor after the bacteria have left the gastric mucosa [121, 122]. Moreover, H+/K+ ATPase autoantibodies, which are closely linked to classical autoimmune gastritis, are also important indicators of mucosal atrophy in *H. pylori* chronic gastritis [123]. *H. pylori* also disappears from the gastric mucosa as a result of the histological and physiological changes induced by chronic atrophy in the case of gastric cancer [124].

Infection with *H. pylori* can also cause malabsorption of different micronutrients [125] like vitamin $B_{12}$ [125-127]. A systematic review and meta-analysis of 17 studies with 2454 patients demonstrated a significant reduction in serum vitamin $B_{12}$ levels in patients infected with *H. pylori* when compared with uninfected persons [128]. Marino et al. demonstrated a correlation between the decrease in serum vitamin $B_{12}$ levels and the increase in serum homocysteine due to *H. pylori* infection in 62 older patients: in these same patients, following infection eradication, an increase in serum vitamin $B_{12}$ levels and a decrease in serum homocysteine levels occurred until normalization was reached [127].

The intimately association of pernicious anemia with the probability to develop stomach cancer was widely recognized by scientific community many years before the relationship between *H. pylori* and stomach cancer was known [129-132]. Recently, Vanella et al. validated this association through a systematic review and meta-analysis, establishing that patients with pernicious anemia (vitamin $B_{12}$ deficiency) have a relative risk of developing gastric cancer of 6.8 (95% CI: 2.6–18.1) [133].

### *2.2.2. Pathophysiology of vitamin $B_{12}$ deficiency*

The pathophysiological mechanism by which *H. pylori* is related to the etiology of vitamin $B_{12}$ deficiency has not been fully clarified, and many questions remain. Possible explanations aiming to clarify the association of *H. pylori* with vitamin $B_{12}$ deficiency are described below. It is not yet known why this association occurs in some patients but not in others, where a different association is presented or the course of the infection is asymptomatic, as happens in most cases [78].

Vitamin $B_{12}$ deficiency manifests as antibodies against intrinsic factor and the parietal cells in the stomach, achlorhydria, and decreased pepsinogen I and gastrin, thereby presenting an histological picture of chronic type A gastritis (autoimmune) [105]. The lack of intrinsic factor, which occurs as result of these changes in the gastric mucosa, reduces the absorption and transport of vitamin $B_{12}$ that comes from the diet. Chronic atrophic gastritis, induced immunologically, evolves over a period of 10–30 years, until reaching gastric atrophy and the development of pernicious anemia, to the extent that the stores of vitamin $B_{12}$ are depleted [105]. Vitamin $B_{12}$ deficiency, parallel to the development of pernicious anemia, causes peripheral neuropathy and lesions in the posterior and lateral columns of the spinal cord, known as subacute combined degeneration, that progresses with demyelination and axial degeneration and eventually neural death [105].

### *2.2.3. Management of vitamin $B_{12}$ deficiency in the post-Helicobacter era*

Respect to the management of vitamin $B_{12}$ deficiency in the post-*Helicobacter* era, it must be clarified that *H. pylori* is not the only cause of vitamin $B_{12}$ deficiency, and its incorporation into the consensus and management guidelines of *H. pylori* as an indication to investigate and eradicate the infection is not a substitute for an adequate study of the most common causes of vitamin $B_{12}$ deficiency. These situations are particular to each region, according to the prevalence of vitamin $B_{12}$ deficiency and *H. pylori* infection, which vary from place to place.

A recent systematic review and meta-analysis with the aim of clarifying the association between *H. pylori* and the vitamin $B_{12}$ deficiency evaluated the serum vitamin $B_{12}$ levels from 17 studies involving a total of 2454 patients, infected or not with *H. pylori*. This study revealed that serum vitamin $B_{12}$ levels are significantly lower in infected patients than in uninfected patients and that *H. pylori* eradication significantly increases vitamin $B_{12}$ levels [128]. This has enabled the inclusion of vitamin $B_{12}$ deficiency in the consensus and management guides of *H. pylori* infection as an indication to evaluate and eradicate the bacteria [27, 29].

Before initiating treatment for a patient with vitamin $B_{12}$ deficiency, an assessment of the prevalence of *H. pylori* infection should be performed according to region. Generally, the prevalence is low in developed countries; in these cases should proceed with conventional management of vitamin $B_{12}$ deficiency [134]. In developing countries, the rate of *H. pylori* infection is high; these cases or when the patient, despite living in a country where infection rates are low, comes from a country where the infection rates are high, it should proceed to determine the status of *H. pylori* through a non-invasive test, ideally the $^{13}$C-urea breath test [27]. If the patient is negative for *H. pylori*, it is necessary to investigate other causes of the vitamin $B_{12}$ deficiency and treat the patient conventionally [134], whereas if the patient is positive for *H. pylori*, it is indispensable to eradicate the infection [27].

After 6–8 weeks of the treatment, the infection eradication must be confirmed using a non-invasive test, ideally with $^{13}$C-urea breath test [27]. If eradication is not achieved, it is mandatory to establish a new therapy scheme until eradication is achieved. Once *H. pylori* eradication is achieved and an improvement in hematological parameters and vitamin $B_{12}$ levels (complete or partial remission) is obtained, it is important to evaluate them for a certain time. If there is no response, it must establish a conventional management of vitamin $B_{12}$ deficiency [134].

Figure 2 shows a diagnostic and management algorithm of vitamin $B_{12}$ deficiency in the post-*Helicobacter* era, taking into account the prevalence of the infection and *H. pylori* status.

### 2.3. Immune thrombocytopenia (ITP)

ITP is the most frequent immunological disease in hematology [135]. The annual incidence of ITP is 5.5 per 100000 persons when the platelet count cut-off point is $100 \times 10^9$/L and 3.2 per 100000 persons when the platelet count cut-off point is $50 \times 10^9$/L [136]. The chronic form of ITP increases with age, being twice as high in people older than 60 years with respect to those younger than 60 years [136, 137], with a higher incidence in women (2:1) than in men (3:1) [138].

Primary ITP, formerly known as idiopathic thrombocytopenic purpura (ITP) and autoimmune thrombocytopenic purpura, has recently been redefined and adjusted in light of new knowledge represented in the Vicenza Consensus [139]. ITP was established as an autoimmune disorder characterized by isolated thrombocytopenia (peripheral blood platelet count below $100 \times 10^9$/L) in the absence of another possible causes or conditions related to thrombocytopenia [139]. Primary ITP diagnosis continues to be one of the exclusions due to current lack of robust

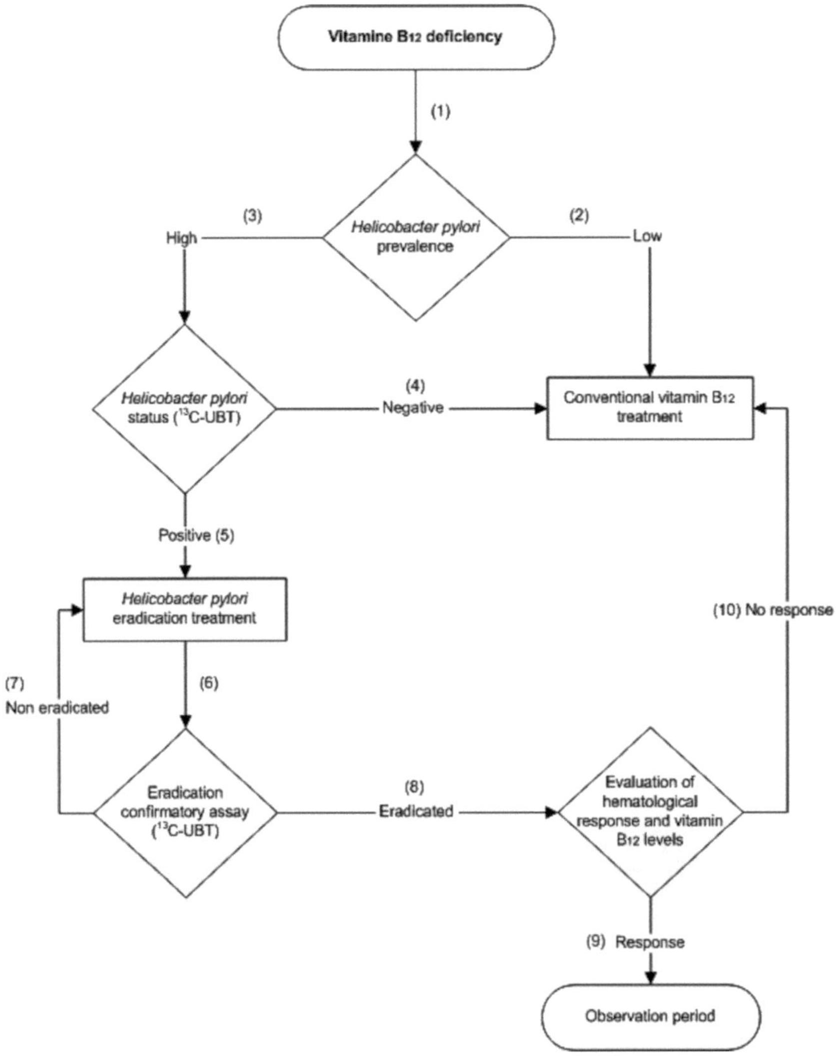


**Figure 2.** Algorithm for the study and management of vitamin $B_{12}$ deficiency in the post-*Helicobacter* era. (1) Before initiating treatment for a patient with vitamin $B_{12}$ deficiency, an assessment of the prevalence of *H. pylori* infection should be performed in each region. Generally, prevalence is high in developing countries and low in developed countries [1]. (2) If the rates of *H. pylori* infection are low, proceed with a conventional management of vitamin $B_{12}$ deficiency [134]. (3) If the rates of *H. pylori* infection are high or the patient, despite living in a country where infection rates are low, comes from a country where the infection rates are high, proceed to determine the status of *H. pylori* through a non-invasive test, ideally the $^{13}$C-urea breath test ($^{13}$C-BUT) [27]. (4) If the patient is negative for *H. pylori*, investigate other causes of vitamin $B_{12}$ deficiency and treat conventionally [134]. (5) If the patient is positive for *H. pylori*, proceed with eradication of the infection [27]. (6) Confirm infection eradication 6–8 weeks after treatment using a non-invasive test, ideally the $^{13}$C-urea breath test [27]. (7) If eradication is not achieved, establish a new scheme of eradication therapy until it is achieved. (8) Once *H. pylori* eradication is achieved, (9) if a response is obtained in the hematological parameters and the serum levels of vitamin $B_{12}$ and homocysteine (complete or partial remission), periodically evaluate the clinical hematological parameters and indicators of vitamin $B_{12}$. (10) If there is no response, proceed with a conventional management of vitamin $B_{12}$ deficiency [134].

clinical and laboratory parameters, with high accuracy to establish its diagnosis [139]. The main clinical concern of primary ITP is the elevated risk of bleeding; however, bleeding symptoms are not present all the time [139].

*H. pylori* infection is included as a new disease at the list of diseases potentially associated with the development of ITP; therefore, it must be ruled out in cases where thrombocytopenia by *H. pylori* infection is suspected [139], according to the establishment by the British Society for Haematology at beginning of 2003 [140]. In addition, the Vicenza Consensus conserved the acronym ITP to refer to the disease itself to avoid confusion and chose the term "primary immune thrombocytopenia" or "primary ITP" as a substitute name for ITP (idiopathic thrombocytopenic purpura) or autoimmune thrombocytopenic purpura, referring to cases where any associated causes are excluded. For cases where an underlying disease is present, it is recommended to use the term "secondary immune thrombocytopenia" or "secondary ITP," followed by the name of the associated condition. For example, for the cases possibly initiated by *H. pylori* infection, it must be used with the extent "secondary ITP *H. pylori*–associated," which required the demonstration of complete resolution of ITP after proving the eradication of the bacteria. This form in clinical practice could be called "ITP *H. pylori*–associated" [139].

### *2.3.1. H. pylori and immune thrombocytopenia*

The association of *H. pylori* with ITP was first reported by Garcia-Perez et al. in Spain in 1993; this report described a patient whose platelet count returned to normal values after eradication of *H. pylori* [141]. The medical literature subsequently reported similar cases in Japan [142-146], Italy [147-149], and Turkey [150].

In Italy, in 1998, Gasbarrini et al. presented the first series of cases demonstrating the association of *H. pylori* with adult ITP, reporting a recovery in platelet counts with disappearance of autoantibodies against platelets in six of eight ITP patients infected with *H. pylori*, after successful eradication of the bacteria [151]. Including this first series [151], 40 series have been described in the medical literature until now, and these reports consistently demonstrate the association between *H. pylori* infection and platelet count recovery following eradication. Ten of these series were reported in Europe: eight in Italy [151-158], one in Turkey [159], and one in Serbia [160], with a total of 495 ITP patients, 288 (58.2%) of whom were infected with *H. pylori*. Of these, 242 received eradication therapy. Successful eradication was achieved in 222 (91.7%) patients, and a platelet response was observed in 108 (48.6%) patients. Asian countries have provided 28 published series: 23 in Japan [161-183], two in China [184, 185], two in Iran [186, 187], and one in South Korea [188], with 1525 total ITP patients, 1089 (71.4%) of whom were infected with *H. pylori*. A total of 929 patients received eradication therapy, it was successful in 811 (87.3%) and 472 (58.2%) patients demonstrated a platelet response. In America, only two series have reported an association between *H. pylori* and ITP: the first in Colombia [189] and the second in Canada [190]. The series in Colombia presented 32 patients with ITP, 29 (90.6%) of whom were infected with *H. pylori*. Those 29 patients received eradication therapy, and it was successful in 26 (89.7%) and 21 (80.8%) patients demonstrated a platelet response [189]. The association of *H. pylori* infection with ITP has not been reported in adults or children from Oceania or the continent of Africa.

A consolidated analysis of the 40 series reported worldwide reveals a total of 2074 patients with ITP, 1410 (68.0%) of whom are *H. pylori*-positive. A total of 1204 received eradication therapy, which succeeded in 1062 (88.2%); 604 (56.9%) of these patients demonstrated a platelet response. In general, Europe has a mean infection rate of 59.2% in patients with ITP and a mean platelet response in 48.6% of those patients; respective rates in Asia are 70.7% and 58.2%, and those in America (Colombia) are 90.6% and 80.8%. When consolidated, the 40 series exhibit a mean infection rate of 68.0% in patients with ITP, with a mean platelet response in 56.9% of those patients [191]. Table 2 summarizes the results of these series demonstrating an association between *H. pylori* infection and ITP development in adults and its response to *H. pylori* eradication [191]. Nevertheless, additional studies in Spain [192], France [193], the United States [193, 194], and Mexico [195] found no association between *H. pylori* infection and adult chronic ITP, explainable, at least in part, by the low prevalence of infection in these countries and insufficient samples.

| Continent | Number of series | Number of patients with ITP | Number of *H. pylori*- infected ITP patients (%) | Number of treated patients | Number *H. pylori*- eradicated patients (%) | Number of patients with platelet response (%) |
|---|---|---|---|---|---|---|
| Europe | 10 [151-160] | 495 | 288 (58.2) | 242 | 222 (91.7) | 108 (48.6) |
| Asia | 28 [161-188] | 1525 | 1089 (71.4) | 929 | 811 (87.3) | 472 (58.2) |
| America | 2 [189, 190] | 54 | 33 (90.6) | 33 | 29 (87.9) | 24 (82.8) |
| Worldwide total | 40 [151-190] | 2074 | 1410 (68.0) | 1204 | 1062 (88.2) | 604 (56.9) |

*Source*: Modified from Campuzano et al. [191]

**Table 2.** *Helicobacter pylori* and immune thrombocytopenia in adults

Regarding to the association of *H. pylori* infection with ITP in children, it is important to clarify that childhood ITP has a different course than ITP in adults [135]. The few studies that have thus far addressed the relationship between ITP and *H. pylori* in children are contradictory: certain groups in China [196], Japan [197], Iran [198], Finland [199], Netherlands [200], and Italy [201, 202] have identified an association between infection and ITP in children, with platelet count recovery in an average of 35.2% of the patients [191]. This rate is much lower than the response rate observed in adult patients with ITP, which is greater than 50% [151-190]. Meanwhile, other groups in Turkey [203], Italy [204, 205], Thailand [206], and Hungary [207] found no association and the response to eradication ranged from none [203, 204, 208] to very poor [205, 207].

### *2.3.2. Pathophysiology of secondary ITP (associated with H. pylori infection)*

The origin of primary ITP is associated with congenital or acquired immune changes that lead to an immune system response against platelets or megakaryocytes that cannot be attributed to other causal changes. In secondary ITP, alternative primary events are identified that lead to the development of this autoimmune response [209]. In the case of *H. pylori* as causal agent of this disease, several mechanisms have been described that contribute to the development of the autoimmune response. One of these mechanisms is a change in the balance of Fcγ receptors, involved in the activation of monocytes, and their relation to the inhibitory Fc receptor FcγRIIB. *H. pylori* infection decreases the levels of FcγRIIB, leading to increased activated monocytes through Fcγ receptors, with elevated non-specific phagocytosis, resulting in overactivation of B and T lymphocytes. These results were confirmed by reversing monocyte activation following *H. pylori* eradication treatment, with reducing generation of autoantibodies by B lymphocytes and overactivation of innate and acquired autoimmune response, and increasing the amount of circulating platelets [179].

In conjunction with the overeactivation of monocytes, autoantibody production has also been described in ITP, which can opsonize the platelets and induce antibody-mediated phagocytosis by the reticuloendothelial system in the spleen. This response is attributed to molecular mimicry of infection-related bacterial proteins. The principal antigens associated with the autoimmune response against the platelets include the amino acid sequences of virulence factors such as VacA, CagA [17, 178] and urease B, which are present during *H. pylori* infection [210]. The similarities shared between these antigens and platelet surface glycoproteins, like the glycoprotein IIIa among other platelet antigens not yet identified, are associated with anti-CagA antibody production [178] and demonstrate the importance of *H. pylori* infection in ITP.

#### *2.3.3. Management of ITP in the post-Helicobacter era*

Concerning to the management of ITP in the post-*Helicobacter* era, it is important to clarify that *H. pylori* is not the only cause of thrombocytopenia, and although the indication, investigation, and treatment of infection should be considered, it is no substitute for an adequate study of the etiologies more frequently associated with thrombocytopenia, which are particular to each region. The 40 series of cases previously discussed, a meta-analysis [211] and two systematic reviews [212, 213] demonstrated the burden of *H. pylori* infection on the development of ITP and that eradicating the infection improves the platelet count in more than 50% of the adult patients with chronic ITP [211-213]. This has permitted the scientific community, in particular the consensus and management guides of *H. pylori* infection, to include ITP as an indication for evaluating and eradicating the infection prior to proceeding with other traditional interventions in both adults and children [21, 23-30].

The American Society of Hematology (ASH) recognized *H. pylori* as a new cause of ITP and established to investigate and eradicate the bacteria during the basic evaluation of patients before applying conventional treatments for the disease [209]. In addition, the International Working Group for standardization of terminology, definitions and outcome criteria in immune thrombocytopenic purpura of adults and children, of the same Society, created a new ITP-associated group denominated "secondary ITP *H. pylori*–associated" [139]. Likewise, since 2003, the British Society for Haematology incorporated the study and eradication of *H. pylori* into their ITP management guidelines [140].

Before initiating treatment for a patient with ITP, an assessment of the prevalence of *H. pylori* infection should be performed according to the region. Generally, the prevalence is low in developed countries; these cases should proceed with conventional management of ITP

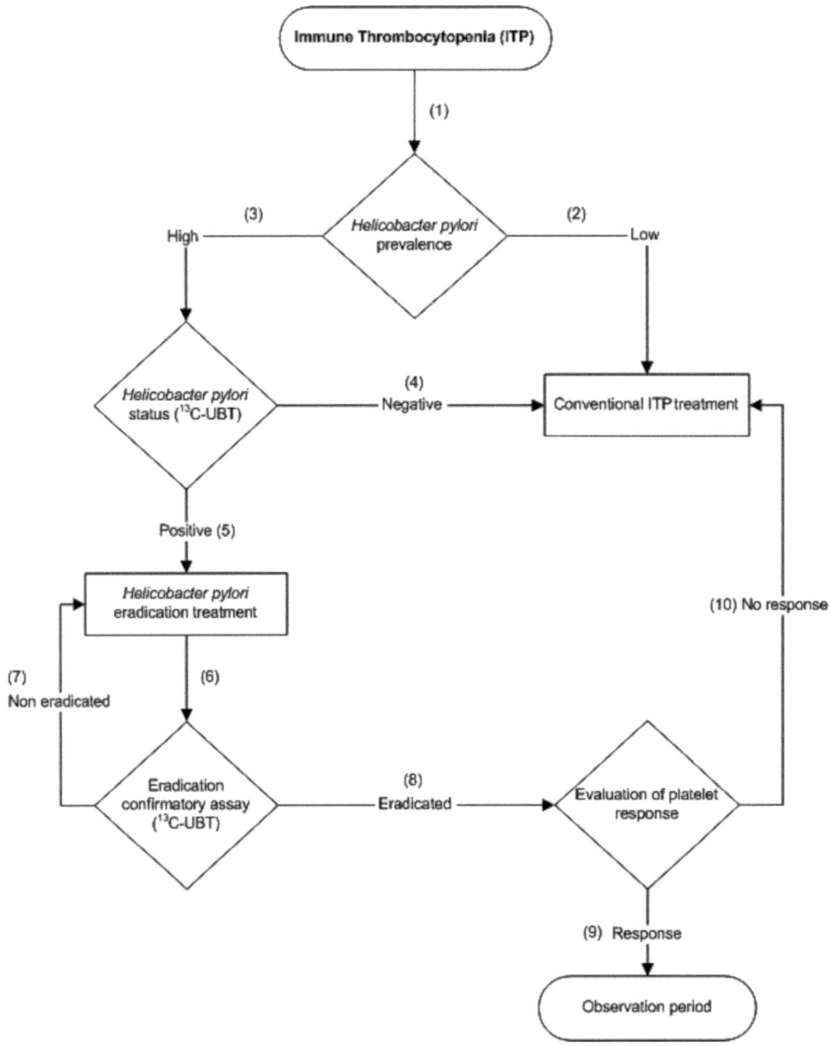


**Figure 3.** Algorithm for the study and management of immune thrombocytopenia (ITP) in the post-*Helicobacter* era. (1) Before initiating treatment for a patient with ITP, an assessment of the prevalence of *H. pylori* infection should be performed in each region. Generally, prevalence is high in developing countries and low in developed countries [1]. (2) If the rates of *H. pylori* infection are low, proceed with a conventional management of ITP [140, 209]. (3) If the rates of *H. pylori* infection are high or the patient, despite living in a country where infection rates are low, comes from a country where the infection rates are high, proceed to determine the status of *H. pylori* through a non-invasive test, ideally a $^{13}$C-urea breath test ($^{13}$C-BUT) [27]. (4) If the patient is negative for *H. pylori*, investigate other causes of thrombocytopenia and treat conventionally [140, 209]. (5) If the patient is positive for *H. pylori*, proceed with eradication of the infection [27]. (6) Confirm infection eradication 6–8 weeks after treatment using a non-invasive test, ideally a $^{13}$C-urea breath test [27]. (7) If eradication is not achieved, establish a new scheme of eradication therapy and continue treatment until it is achieved. (8) Once *H. pylori* eradication is achieved, (9) if a platelet response is obtained (complete or partial remission), periodically evaluate the platelet count. (10) If there is no platelet response, proceed with a conventional management of ITP [140, 209]. Reprinted from "Proof of an association between *Helicobacter pylori* and idiopathic thrombocytopenic purpura in Latin America" by G. Campuzano-Maya, 2007, *Helicobacter*, 12, p. 270. Copyright 1999–2015 by John Wiley & Sons, Inc. Reprinted with author permission [189].

[140, 209]. In developing countries, the rate of *H. pylori* infection is high; in these cases or when the patient, despite living in a country where infection rates are low, comes from a country where the infection rates are high, it should proceed to determine the status of *H. pylori* through a non-invasive test, ideally the $^{13}$C-urea breath test [27]. If the patient is negative for *H. pylori*, it is necessary to investigate other causes of thrombocytopenia and treat the patient conventionally [140, 209], whereas if the patient is positive for *H. pylori* it is indispensable to eradicate the infection [27].

After 6–8 weeks of treatment, the infection eradication must be confirmed using a non-invasive test, ideally with $^{13}$C-urea breath test [27]. If eradication is not achieved, it is mandatory to establish a new therapy scheme until eradication is achieved. Once *H. pylori* eradication is achieved and obtained a platelet response (complete or partial remission), it is important to periodically evaluate platelet count. If there is no platelet response, it must establish a conventional management of ITP [140, 209].

Figure 3 shows a diagnostic and management algorithm for ITP in the post-*Helicobacter* era, taking into account the prevalence and status of *H. pylori* infection [189].

## 3. Hematological diseases not recognized as related to *H. pylori*

This group includes autoimmune neutropenia, antiphospholipid syndrome, Henoch–Schönlein purpura, plasma cell dyscrasias, such as monoclonal gammopathy of undetermined significance (MGUS) and multiple myeloma, and other diseases possibly associated or implicated, such as leukemia and hemorrhagic manifestations with hematologic origin, like congenital and acquired coagulopathies and anticoagulation.

### 3.1. Immune neutropenia

This association was first proposed in 2002 by Gupta et al. in England, who reported the case of a patient with neutropenia (400 neutrophils/μL) that rapidly returned to normal values following the eradication of *H. pylori* infection [214]. Since then, two new studies have been reported, which include eight and 69 patients [215, 216] and coincide with the original report of Gupta et al. [214]. In the future, it is recommended that in patients with neutropenia that is suspected of being immunological the *H. pylori* status be established and proceed to eradicate if positive [214] as part of good medical practice.

### 3.2. Antiphospholipid syndrome

Similarly to immune neutropenia, antiphospholipid syndrome, a coagulation disorder of immunologic origin characterized by both arterial and venous thrombosis and associated with pregnancy complications, such as abortion, premature childbirth, and pre-eclampsia [217], was proposed as an extragastric association of *H. pylori* infection in 2001 by Cicconi et al. in Italy. These authors reported the case of a woman in whom antiphospholipid syndrome disappeared after the eradication of *H. pylori* infection [218]. At the moment, there are no new reports of this association in the medical literature possibly only because it is not being considered or investigated. However, it is worth recalling that antiphospholipid syndrome has been associated with other diseases of immunologic origin that in turn are associated with *H. pylori* infection, such as ITP [189, 219, 220], systemic lupus erythematosus [221], and central serous chorioretinitis [222, 223].

### 3.3. Henoch–Schönlein purpura

Henoch–Schönlein purpura is an immunologic disease of unknown etiology manifested by small vessel leukocytoclastic vasculitis with deposits of immunoglobulin A (IgA) in the skin, joints, gastrointestinal tract, and kidneys [224]. Henoch–Schönlein purpura is included in this review because it is part of the differential diagnosis of thrombocytopenia, particularly ITP discussed previously, which manifests as purpuric lesions on the skin. The association of *H. pylori* with Henoch–Schönlein purpura was proposed in the case of a 21-year-old man by Rainauer et al. in Germany in 1996 [225]. Since then, many studies have confirmed the association in adults [226-231], children, and adolescents [229, 232, 233], with the disappearance of clinical manifestations in *H. pylori*-positive cases after eradication [229-231].

### 3.4. Plasma cell dyscrasias

Plasma cell dyscrasias are among the most frequent clonal diseases in elderly persons and include MGUS, multiple myeloma, solitary plasmacytoma, plasma cell leukemia, Waldenström's macroglobulinemia, and other chronic myeloproliferative syndromes of B lymphocytes [234]. Plasma cell dyscrasias may present an asymptomatic course or pass from one disease to another; for example, MGUS, a completely benign and asymptomatic condition that does not require treatment, can transform into a more severe and potentially fatal disease, such as multiple myeloma [234].

The association of plasma cell dyscrasias with stomach diseases has been known for many years, before the discovery that the stomach could be colonized by bacteria [3]. Gastrointestinal plasmacytomas were documented by the father of modern medicine, Sir William Osler, in 1920 [235], and for many years, the association of these and multiple myeloma with pernicious anemia [236, 237] and gastric cancer [238-242], entities clearly correlated with *H. pylori* infection, has been known. Perhaps, the most important evidence of the association of *H. pylori* infection with plasma cell dyscrasias is that some plasmacytomas disappear after the eradication of *H. pylori*. The authors who have analyzed this facet of infection by *H. pylori* have agreed to recommending that in all patients with these manifestations be offered the opportunity of evaluated and eradicate the infection if present [243-245]. Other associations described include a clear interaction between MALT lymphoma of the stomach and MGUS [246] as well as Waldenström's disease and MALT [247].

The relation of multiple myeloma with gastric MALT type lymphomas [248-254] was identified many years before *H. pylori* was known. Today, it is known that in MALT lymphoma, *H. pylori* antigens can also stimulate plasma cells. The plasmacytomas discussed previously could be the expression of a localized myeloma, and once disseminated, it would not be possible to differentiate one from another. Wöhrer at al. have shown an association of gastric lymphomas with gastric myelomas [255]; besides, they described a case of plasmacytoma of the orbit, which completely remitted after the eradication of *H. pylori* [256]. Therefore, it is logical that all patients with a disease diagnosis related to plasma cells should be studied for *H. pylori* and if positive, be treated with eradication therapy prior to starting conventional treatment.

According to Malik et al., MGUS, important in the study of patients with plasma cell dyscrasia, may be related to *H. pylori* as result of chronic antigenic stimulation of B lymphocytes in the gastric mucosa by the bacteria. Resolution of the gammopathy is observed in up to 30% of cases by eradicating the bacteria [257], a relationship confirmed by some authors [246, 258] but not by others [215, 259].

### 3.5. Other hematologic manifestations

According to the medical literature, other hematologic manifestations demonstrate possible associations with *H. pylori* infection, which despite the low abundance of information entailed important clinical implications. Lehtine et al. reported that in Iceland, anti-*H. pylori* immunoglobulin G was associated with increased risk of childhood leukemia in offspring (OR = 2.8, 95% CI: 1.1–6.9), whereas in Finland, it is not associated. Because anti-*H. pylori* immunoglobulin G indicates chronic carriage of the bacteria, early colonization of the offspring probably differs between Iceland and Finland, two affluent countries [260]. This type of study should be replicated at other sites, especially those where the prevalence of *H. pylori* is high, such as in Asian countries and Latin America. Diamantidis et al. reported that although there is no evidence for a causal relationship between *H. pylori* infection and myelodysplastic syndrome (MDS), an increased prevalence of *H. pylori* infection among MDS patients has been found. This is an interesting finding that deserves further investigation because it may indicate a common factor causing susceptibilities to both MDS and *H. pylori* infection or that *H. pylori* might influence the pathophysiology of MDS [261]. Recently, Kawamata et al. described the case of a patient with *H. pylori*-induced thrombocytosis clinically indistinguishable from essential thrombocythemia, which disappeared after the eradication of the infection [262].

Another problem emerging in clinical practice is the inherent increased risk of hemorrhage in patients with hematologic diseases; *H. pylori*, according to preliminary studies, would be a risk factor for the occurrence of these events. This is the case for patients with acute leukemia who are infected with *H. pylori*: the risk of gastrointestinal hemorrhaging during treatment is greater than in non-infected patients. This would be reduced if all patients with leukemia are offered the screening and eradication of *H. pylori* when treatment begins [263]. In patients with potentially hemorrhagic diseases, such as hemophilia (A and B) and von Willebrand's disease, *H. pylori* infection should be considered as an important cause of upper gastrointestinal bleeding. It is recommended a stool antigen test as a new and non-invasive screening test for diagnosis of *H. pylori* infection in all patients with hereditary hemorrhagic disorders [264]. These procedures are cost efficient for the health system, if one takes into account that the screening, followed by treatment of all infected patients, yields a reduction of direct costs over a 5-year period of 130 US$ per screened patient [265]. Therefore, due to increased bleeding complications, *H. pylori* screening and therapy appear mandatory in patients with bleeding disorders [266]. This conduct would also be applicable for patients undergoing prophylactic anticoagulation therapy [267] like aspirin [95]. The study and eradication of *H. pylori* in patients with chronic idiopathic neutropenia are also suggested, wherein splenomegaly, it is probably associated with *H. pylori,* as evidenced by correlation between splenic volume and infection period [215, 216].

## 4. Conclusions

The recognition of hematologic diseases associated with *H. pylori* infection and its incorporation as an indication for study and eradication in the consensus and management guides for *H. pylori* infection represent a profound paradigm shift in the management of these diseases and a great advance for humanity. In addition to the benefits that eradication brings to the infected people, especially those related to gastric cancer [4] and peptic ulcer disease [3], the paradigm shifts introduced into medical practice and the medico-social impact expected from these new paradigms are summarized in the following paragraphs.

### 4.1. Iron deficiency

The management of iron deficiency is palliative and based on iron supplementation [32], where there is often no impact on the direct cause associated with ferropenia [35]. With the incorporation of iron deficiency, with or without anemia, into the consensus and management guides for *H. pylori* infection as an indication to investigate and eradicate the bacteria [21-30], a new paradigm was generated, where the etiology of ferropenia can be infectious and the eradication of *H. pylori* may be sufficient to cure the deficiency, in the strict sense of the word [46-50]. Under the new paradigm, where eradication of the infection corrects the iron deficiency, in addition to restoring health [46-50] and increasing productivity [32], the prevalence of *H. pylori* infection and the diseases associated with it, such as gastric cancer [4] and gastric acid disease [3], decreases.

### 4.2. Vitamin $B_{12}$ deficiency

The management of vitamin $B_{12}$ deficiency is also palliative and based on vitamin supplementation, where there is little impact on the initial cause of the deficiency [134]. With the incorporation of vitamin $B_{12}$ deficiency into the consensus and management guides for *H. pylori* infection as an indication to investigate and eradicate the bacteria [27, 29], a new paradigm was generated, where the etiology of vitamin $B_{12}$ deficiency can be infectious and the eradication of *H. pylori* may be sufficient to correct it [127]. Under this new paradigm, where eradication of infection corrects the vitamin $B_{12}$ deficiency by a curative rather than palliative treatment [127], the patient is released from a chronic disease [134] closely related to gastric cancer and from diverse diseases such as Alzheimer's disease [107, 108], depression [111], stroke [112, 113], pulmonary embolism [114], acute myocardial infarction, and coronary heart disease [116], which are regulated through homocysteine and generate high morbidity, mortality, and costs for health systems.

### 4.3. Immune thrombocytopenia

The treatment of ITP is palliative, not curative, and is oriented toward controlling the production of antibodies against platelets using medication or through the removal of organs that sequester platelets, such as the spleen [140, 209]. With the incorporation of ITP into the consensus and management guides for *H. pylori* infection as an indication to investigate and eradicate the bacteria [21, 23-30], a new paradigm was generated, where the etiology of ITP can be infectious and the eradication of *H. pylori* may be sufficient to cure it, in the strict sense of the word [151-190]. Under the new paradigm, where the eradication of infection leads to correction of the platelet count with definitive cure of ITP, the patient is freed from a chronic disease [140, 209] by a curative rather than palliative treatment [151-190]. Furthermore, the eradication of the infection in these patients reduces the prevalence of gastric cancer and peptic acid disease, with which it is closely related and which contribute to high morbidity, mortality, and costs for health systems.

## Acknowledgements

The author gratefully acknowledges to Verónica Tangarife-Castaño for her insightful discussions and help with the English translation as well as the willingness and collaboration.

## Author details

Germán Campuzano-Maya*

Address all correspondence to: gcm@lch.co

Group of Clinical Pathology, Laboratorio Clínico Hematológico®, Faculty of Medicine, Universidad de Antioquia, Medellín, Colombia

## References

[1] Pounder RE, Ng D. The prevalence of *Helicobacter pylori* infection in different countries. Aliment Pharmacol Ther. 1995; 9 Suppl 2: 33–39.

[2] EUROGAST Study Group. Epidemiology of, and risk factors for, *Helicobacter pylori* infection among 3194 asymptomatic subjects in 17 populations. Gut 1993; 34: 1672–1676.

[3] Warren JR, Marshall B. Unidentified curved baccilli on gastric epithelium in active chronic gastritis. Lancet 1983; 1:1273-1275.

[4] Correa P. Gastric cancer: overview. Gastroenterol Clin North Am. 2013; 42: 211–217. DOI: 10.1016/j.gtc.2013.01.002.

[5] Stolte M, Bayerdorffer E, Morgner A, Alpen B, Wundisch T, Thiede C, et al. Helicobacter and gastric MALT lymphoma. Gut 2002; 50 Suppl 3: III19–III24.

[6] Gasbarrini A, Franceschi F, Armuzzi A, Ojetti V, Candelli M, Torre ES, et al. Extradigestive manifestations of *Helicobacter pylori* gastric infection. Gut 1999; 45 Suppl 1: I9–I12.

[7] Realdi G, Dore MP, Fastame L. Extradigestive manifestations of *Helicobacter pylori* infection: fact and fiction. Dig Dis Sci. 1999; 44: 229–236.

[8] Carloni E, Cremonini F, Di Caro S, Padalino C, Gerardino L, Santoliquido A, et al. *Helicobacter pylori*-related extradigestive diseases and effects of eradication therapy. Dig Liver Dis. 2000; 32 Suppl 3: S214–S216.

[9] De Koster E, De Bruyne I, Langlet P, Deltenre M. Evidence based medicine and extradigestive manifestations of *Helicobacter pylori*. Acta Gastroenterol Belg. 2000; 63: 388–392.

[10] Sherman PM, Lin FY. Extradigestive manifestation of *Helicobacter pylori* infection in children and adolescents. Can J Gastroenterol. 2005; 19: 421–424.

[11] Solnick JV, Franceschi F, Roccarina D, Gasbarrini A. Extragastric manifestations of *Helicobacter pylori* infection—other Helicobacter species. Helicobacter 2006; 11 Suppl 1: 46–51.

[12] Bohr UR, Annibale B, Franceschi F, Roccarina D, Gasbarrini A. Extragastric manifestations of *Helicobacter pylori* infection — other Helicobacters. Helicobacter 2007; 12 Suppl 1: 45–53.

[13] Moyaert H, Franceschi F, Roccarina D, Ducatelle R, Haesebrouck F, Gasbarrini A. Extragastric manifestations of *Helicobacter pylori* infection: other Helicobacters. Helicobacter 2008; 13 Suppl 1: 47–57. DOI: 10.1111/j.1523-5378.2008.00634.x.

[14] Pellicano R, Franceschi F, Saracco G, Fagoonee S, Roccarina D, Gasbarrini A. Helicobacters and extragastric diseases. Helicobacter 2009; 14 Suppl 1: 58–68. DOI: 10.1111/j.1523-5378.2009.00699.x.

[15] Figura N, Franceschi F, Santucci A, Bernardini G, Gasbarrini G, Gasbarrini A. Extragastric manifestations of *Helicobacter pylori* infection. Helicobacter 2010; 15 Suppl 1: 60–68. DOI: 10.1111/j.1523-5378.2010.00778.x.

[16] Suzuki H, Franceschi F, Nishizawa T, Gasbarrini A. Extragastric manifestations of *Helicobacter pylori* infection. Helicobacter 2011; 16 Suppl 1: 65–69. DOI: 10.1111/j.1523-5378.2011.00883.x.

[17] Banic M, Franceschi F, Babic Z, Gasbarrini A. Extragastric manifestations of *Helicobacter pylori* infection. Helicobacter 2012; 17 Suppl 1: 49–55. DOI: 10.1111/j.1523-5378.2012.00983.x.

[18] Roubaud Baudron C, Franceschi F, Salles N, Gasbarrini A. Extragastric diseases and *Helicobacter pylori*. Helicobacter 2013; 18 Suppl 1: 44–51. DOI: 10.1111/hel.12077.

[19] Pacifico L, Osborn JF, Tromba V, Romaggioli S, Bascetta S, Chiesa C. *Helicobacter pylori* infection and extragastric disorders in children: a critical update. World J Gastroenterol. 2014; 20: 1379–1401. DOI: 10.3748/wjg.v20.i6.1379.

[20] Al Sayed A, Anand PS, Kamath KP, Patil S, Preethanath RS, Anil S. Oral cavity as an extragastric reservoir of *Helicobacter pylori*. ISRN Gastroenterol. 2014; 2014: 261369. DOI: 10.1155/2014/261369.

[21] Malfertheiner P, Megraud F, O'Morain C, Bazzoli F, El-Omar E, Graham D, et al. Current concepts in the management of *Helicobacter pylori* infection: the Maastricht III Consensus Report. Gut. 2007; 56: 772–781. DOI: 10.1136/gut.2006.101634.

[22] Chey WD, Wong BC. American College of Gastroenterology guideline on the management of *Helicobacter pylori* infection. Am J Gastroenterol. 2007; 102: 1808–1825.

[23] Caselli M, Zullo A, Maconi G, Parente F, Alvisi V, Casetti T, et al. Cervia II Working Group Report 2006: guidelines on diagnosis and treatment of *Helicobacter pylori* infection in Italy. Dig Liver Dis. 2007; 39: 782–789.

[24] Kim N, Kim JJ, Choe YH, Kim HS, Kim JI, Chung IS. Diagnosis and treatment guidelines for *Helicobacter pylori* infection in Korea. Korean J Gastroenterol. 2009; 54: 269–278.

[25] Fock KM, Katelaris P, Sugano K, Ang TL, Hunt R, Talley NJ, et al. Second Asia–Pacific Consensus Guidelines for *Helicobacter pylori* infection. J Gastroenterol Hepatol. 2009; 24: 1587–1600. DOI: 10.1111/j.1440-1746.2009.05982.x.

[26] Asaka M, Kato M, Takahashi S, Fukuda Y, Sugiyama T, Ota H, et al. Guidelines for the management of *Helicobacter pylori* infection in Japan: 2009 revised edition. Helicobacter 2010; 15: 1–20. DOI: 10.1111/j.1523-5378.2009.00738.x.

[27] Malfertheiner P, Megraud F, O'Morain CA, Atherton J, Axon AT, Bazzoli F, et al. Management of *Helicobacter pylori* infection—the Maastricht IV/Florence Consensus Report. Gut 2012; 61: 646–664. DOI: 10.1136/gutjnl-2012-302084.

[28] Coelho LG, Maguinilk I, Zaterka S, Parente JM, Passos Mdo C, Moraes-Filho JP. 3th Brazilian Consensus on *Helicobacter pylori*. Arq Gastroenterol. 2013; 50: 81–96. DOI: 10.1590/S0004-28032013005000001.

[29] Gisbert JP, Calvet X, Bermejo F, Boixeda D, Bory F, Bujanda L, et al. III Spanish Consensus Conference on *Helicobacter pylori* infection. Gastroenterol Hepatol. 2013; 36: 340–374. DOI: 10.1016/j.gastrohep.2013.01.011.

[30] Liu WZ, Xie Y, Cheng H, Lu NH, Hu FL, Zhang WD, et al. The Fourth Chinese National Consensus Report on the management of *Helicobacter pylori* infection. J Dig Dis. 2013; 104: 516–518. DOI: 10.1111/1751-2980.12034.

[31] Kim SG, Jung HK, Lee HL, Jang JY, Lee H, Kim CG, et al. Guidelines for the diagnosis and treatment of *Helicobacter pylori* infection in Korea, 2013 revised edition. J Gastroenterol Hepatol. 2014; 29: 1371–1386. DOI: 10.1111/jgh.12607.

[32] WHO/UNICEF/UNU. Iron deficiency anemia assessment, prevention, and control. 2001. Available from: http://www.who.int/nutrition/publications/en/ida_assessment_prevention_control.pdf [accessed April 13, 2014].

[33] McLean E, Cogswell M, Egli I, Wojdyla D, de Benoist B. Worldwide prevalence of anaemia, WHO Vitamin and Mineral Nutrition Information System, 1993–2005. Public Health Nutr. 2009; 12: 444–454. DOI: 10.1017/S1368980008002401.

[34] Zimmermann MB, Hurrell RF. Nutritional iron deficiency. Lancet 2007; 370: 511–520. DOI: 10.1016/S0140-6736(07)61235-5.

[35] Goodnough LT, Nemeth E. Iron deficiency and related disorders. In: Greer JP, Arber DA, Glader B, List AF, Means RTJ, Paraskevas F, et al., editors. Wintrobe's Clinical Hematology. 13 Ed. Philadelphia, PA: Lippincott Williams & Wilkins; 2013. p. 617–642.

[36] Blecker U, Renders F, Lanciers S, Vandenplas Y. Syncopes leading to the diagnosis of a *Helicobacter pylori* positive chronic active haemorrhagic gastritis. Eur J Pediatr. 1991; 150: 560–561.

[37] Bruel H, Dabadie A, Pouedras P, Gambert C, Le Gall E, Jezequel C. Revealing acute anemia of *Helicobacter pylori* gastritis. Ann Pediatr (Paris). 1993; 40: 364–367.

[38] Dufour C, Brisigotti M, Fabretti G, Luxardo P, Mori PG, Barabino A. *Helicobacter pylori* gastric infection and sideropenic refractory anemia. J Pediatr Gastroenterol Nutr. 1993; 17: 225–227.

[39] Marignani M, Angeletti S, Bordi C, Malagnino F, Mancino C, Delle Fave G, et al. Reversal of long-standing iron deficiency anaemia after eradication of *Helicobacter pylori* infection. Scand J Gastroenterol. 1997; 32: 617–622.

[40] Milman N, Rosenstock S, Andersen L, Jorgensen T, Bonnevie O. Serum ferritin, hemoglobin, and *Helicobacter pylori* infection: a seroepidemiologic survey comprising 2794 Danish adults. Gastroenterology 1998; 115: 268–274.

[41] Annibale B, Marignani M, Monarca B, Antonelli G, Marcheggiano A, Martino G, et al. Reversal of iron deficiency anemia after *Helicobacter pylori* eradication in patients with asymptomatic gastritis. Ann Intern Med. 1999; 131: 668–672. DOI: 199911020-00006 pii.

[42] Barabino A, Dufour C, Marino CE, Claudiani F, De Alessandri A. Unexplained refractory iron-deficiency anemia associated with *Helicobacter pylori* gastric infection in children: further clinical evidence. J Pediatr Gastroenterol Nutr. 1999; 28: 116–119.

[43] Capurso G, Marignani M, Delle Fave G, Annibale B. Iron-deficiency anemia in premenopausal women: why not consider atrophic body gastritis and *Helicobacter pylori* role? Am J Gastroenterol. 1999; 94: 3084–3085.

[44] Peach HG, Bath NE, Farish SJ. *Helicobacter pylori* infection: an added stressor on iron status of women in the community. Med J Aust. 1998; 169: 188–190.

[45] Collett JA, Burt MJ, Frampton CM, Yeo KH, Chapman TM, Buttimore RC, et al. Seroprevalence of *Helicobacter pylori* in the adult population of Christchurch: risk factors and relationship to dyspeptic symptoms and iron studies. N Z Med J. 1999; 112: 292–295.

[46] Muhsen K, Cohen D. *Helicobacter pylori* infection and iron stores: a systematic review and meta-analysis. Helicobacter 2008; 13: 323–340. DOI: 10.1111/j.1523-5378.2008.00617.x.

[47] Qu XH, Huang XL, Xiong P, Zhu CY, Huang YL, Lu LG, et al. Does *Helicobacter pylori* infection play a role in iron deficiency anemia? A meta-analysis. World J Gastroenterol. 2010; 16: 886–896.

[48] Huang X, Qu X, Yan W, Huang Y, Cai M, Hu B, et al. Iron deficiency anaemia can be improved after eradication of *Helicobacter pylori*. Postgrad Med J. 2010; 86: 272–278. DOI: 10.1136/pgmj.2009.089987.

[49] Yuan W, Li Y, Yang K, Ma B, Guan Q, Wang D, et al. Iron deficiency anemia in *Helicobacter pylori* infection: meta-analysis of randomized controlled trials. Scand J Gastroenterol. 2010; 45: 665–676. DOI: 10.3109/00365521003663670.

[50] Zhang ZF, Yang N, Zhao G, Zhu L, Zhu Y, Wang LX. Effect of *Helicobacter pylori* eradication on iron deficiency. Chin Med J (Engl). 2010; 123: 1924–1930.

[51] Ashorn M, Ruuska T, Makipernaa A. *Helicobacter pylori* and iron deficiency anaemia in children. Scand J Gastroenterol. 2001; 36: 701–705.

[52] Seo JK, Ko JS, Choi KD. Serum ferritin and *Helicobacter pylori* infection in children: a sero-epidemiologic study in Korea. J Gastroenterol Hepatol. 2002; 17: 754–757.

[53] Kostaki M, Fessatou S, Karpathios T. Refractory iron-deficiency anaemia due to silent *Helicobacter pylori* gastritis in children. Eur J Pediatr. 2003; 162: 177–179.

[54] Huang LP, Zhuang ML, Bei GP, Gu CP, Li YH. Clinical study on the relation between *Helicobacter pylori* infection and iron-deficiency anemia in children. Zhonghua Liu Xing Bing Xue Za Zhi. 2004; 25: 458.

[55] Yang YJ, Sheu BS, Lee SC, Yang HB, Wu JJ. Children of *Helicobacter pylori*-infected dyspeptic mothers are predisposed to *H. pylori* acquisition with subsequent iron deficiency and growth retardation. Helicobacter 2005; 10: 249–255.

[56] Gessner BD, Baggett HC, Muth PT, Dunaway E, Gold BD, Feng Z, et al. A controlled, household-randomized, open-label trial of the effect that treatment of *Helicobacter pylori* infection has on iron deficiency in children in rural Alaska. J Infect Dis. 2006; 193: 537–546.

[57] Baggett HC, Parkinson AJ, Muth PT, Gold BD, Gessner BD. Endemic iron deficiency associated with *Helicobacter pylori* infection among school-aged children in Alaska. Pediatrics 2006; 117: e396–e404.

[58] Süoglu OD, Gokce S, Saglam AT, Sokucu S, Saner G. Association of *Helicobacter pylori* infection with gastroduodenal disease, epidemiologic factors and iron-deficiency anemia in Turkish children undergoing endoscopy, and impact on growth. Pediatr Int. 2007; 49: 858–863.

[59] Sarker SA, Mahmud H, Davidsson L, Alam NH, Ahmed T, Alam N, et al. Causal relationship of *Helicobacter pylori* with iron-deficiency anemia or failure of iron supplementation in children. Gastroenterology 2008; 135: 1534–1542. DOI: 10.1053/j.gastro.2008.07.030.

[60] Haghi-Ashtiani MT, Monajemzadeh M, Motamed F, Mahjoub F, Sharifan M, Shahsiah R, et al. Anemia in children with and without *Helicobacter pylori* infection. Arch Med Res. 2008; 39: 536–540. DOI: 10.1016/j.arcmed.2008.04.005.

[61] Choe YH, Lee JE, Kim SK. Effect of *Helicobacter pylori* eradication on sideropenic refractory anaemia in adolescent girls with *Helicobacter pylori* infection. Acta Paediatr. 2000; 89: 154–157.

[62] Choe YH, Kim SK, Hong YC. The relationship between *Helicobacter pylori* infection and iron deficiency: seroprevalence study in 937 pubescent children. Arch Dis Child. 2003; 88: 178.

[63] Hershko C, Hoffbrand AV, Keret D, Souroujon M, Maschler I, Monselise Y, et al. Role of autoimmune gastritis, *Helicobacter pylori* and celiac disease in refractory or unexplained iron deficiency anemia. Haematologica 2005; 90: 585–595.

[64] Parkinson AJ, Gold BD, Bulkow L, Wainwright RB, Swaminathan B, Khanna B, et al. High prevalence of *Helicobacter pylori* in the Alaska native population and association with low serum ferritin levels in young adults. Clin Diagn Lab Immunol. 2000; 7: 885–888.

[65] Berg G, Bode G, Blettner M, Boeing H, Brenner H. *Helicobacter pylori* infection and serum ferritin: a population-based study among 1806 adults in Germany. Am J Gastroenterol. 2001; 96: 1014–1018.

[66] Bini EJ. *Helicobacter pylori* and iron deficiency anemia: guilty as charged? Am J Med. 2001; 111: 495–497.

[67] Cuoco L, Cammarota G, Jorizzo RA, Santarelli L, Cianci R, Montalto M, et al. Link between *Helicobacter pylori* infection and iron-deficiency anaemia in patients with coeliac disease. Scand J Gastroenterol. 2001; 36: 1284–1288.

[68] Choe YH, Kwon YS, Jung MK, Kang SK, Hwang TS, Hong YC. *Helicobacter pylori*-associated iron-deficiency anemia in adolescent female athletes. J Pediatr. 2001; 139: 100–104.

[69] Yoshimura M, Hirai M, Tanaka N, Kasahara Y, Hosokawa O. Remission of severe anemia persisting for over 20 years after eradication of *Helicobacter pylori* in cases of Ménétrier's disease and atrophic gastritis: *Helicobacter pylori* as a pathogenic factor in iron-deficiency anemia. Intern Med. 2003; 42: 971–977.

[70] Nahon S, Lahmek P, Massard J, Lesgourgues B, Mariaud de Serre N, Traissac L, et al. *Helicobacter pylori*-associated chronic gastritis and unexplained iron deficiency anemia: a reliable association? Helicobacter 2003; 8: 573–577.

[71] Ciacci C, Sabbatini F, Cavallaro R, Castiglione F, Di Bella S, Iovino P, et al. *Helicobacter pylori* impairs iron absorption in infected individuals. Dig Liver Dis. 2004; 36: 455–460.

[72] Valiyaveettil AN, Hamide A, Bobby Z, Krishnan R. Effect of anti-*Helicobacter pylori* therapy on outcome of iron-deficiency anemia: a randomized, controlled study. Indian J Gastroenterol. 2005; 24: 155–157.

[73] Cardenas VM, Mulla ZD, Ortiz M, Graham DY. Iron deficiency and *Helicobacter pylori* infection in the United States. Am J Epidemiol. 2006; 163: 127–134.

[74] Chen LH, Luo HS. Effects of H pylori therapy on erythrocytic and iron parameters in iron deficiency anemia patients with *H. pylori*-positive chronic gastristis. World J Gastroenterol. 2007; 13: 5380–5383.

[75] Vijayan G, Sundaram RC, Bobby Z, Hamide A, Selvaraj N, Dasse NR. Increased plasma malondialdehyde and fructosamine in anemic *H. pylori* infected patients: effect of treatment. World J Gastroenterol. 2007; 13: 796–800.

[76] Kaffes A, Cullen J, Mitchell H, Katelaris PH. Effect of *Helicobacter pylori* infection and low-dose aspirin use on iron stores in the elderly. J Gastroenterol Hepatol. 2003; 18: 1024–1028.

[77] Mulayim B, Celik NY, Yanik FF. *Helicobacter pylori* infection detected by C-Urea breath test is associated with iron deficiency anemia in pregnant women. J Obstet Gynaecol Res. 2008; 34: 980–985. DOI: 10.1111/j.1447-0756.2008.00822.x.

[78] Correa P, Piazuelo MB. Natural history of *Helicobacter pylori* infection. Dig Liver Dis. 2008; 40: 490–496. DOI: 10.1016/j.dld.2008.02.035.

[79] Park CH, Valore EV, Waring AJ, Ganz T. Hepcidin, a urinary antimicrobial peptide synthesized in the liver. J Biol Chem. 2001; 276: 7806–7810. DOI: 10.1074/jbc.M008922200.

[80] Kroot JJ, Tjalsma H, Fleming RE, Swinkels DW. Hepcidin in human iron disorders: diagnostic implications. Clin Chem. 2011; 57: 1650–1669. DOI: 10.1373/clinchem.2009.140053.

[81] Cherian S, Forbes DA, Cook AG, Sanfilippo FM, Kemna EH, Swinkels DW, et al. An insight into the relationships between hepcidin, anemia, infections and inflammatory cytokines in pediatric refugees: a cross-sectional study. PLoS One. 2008; 3: e4030. DOI: 10.1371/journal.pone.0004030.

[82] Hershko C, Ronson A. Iron deficiency, Helicobacter infection and gastritis. Acta Haematol. 2009; 122: 97–102. DOI: 10.1159/000243793.

[83] Lee SY, Song EY, Yun YM, Yoon SY, Cho YH, Kim SY, et al. Serum prohepcidin levels in *Helicobacter pylori* infected patients with iron deficiency anemia. Korean J Intern Med. 2010; 25: 195–200. DOI: 10.3904/kjim.2010.25.2.195.

[84] Schwarz P, Kubler JA, Strnad P, Muller K, Barth TF, Gerloff A, et al. Hepcidin is localised in gastric parietal cells, regulates acid secretion and is induced by *Helicobacter pylori* infection. Gut. 2012; 61: 193–201. DOI: 10.1136/gut.2011.241208.

[85] Ozkasap S, Yarali N, Isik P, Bay A, Kara A, Tunc B. The role of prohepcidin in anemia due to *Helicobacter pylori* infection. Pediatr Hematol Oncol. 2013; 30: 425–431. DOI: 10.3109/08880018.2013.783144.

[86] Emiralioglu N, Yenicesu I, Sari S, Egritas O, Poyraz A, Pasaoglu OT, et al. An insight into the relationships between prohepcidin, iron deficiency anemia, and interleukin-6 values in pediatric *Helicobacter pylori* gastritis. Eur J Pediatr. 2015; 174: 903-910. DOI: 10.1007/s00431-014-2482-4.

[87] Sato Y, Yoneyama O, Azumaya M, Takeuchi M, Sasaki SY, Yokoyama J, et al. The relationship between iron deficiency in patients with *Helicobacter pylori*-infected nodular gastritis and the serum prohepcidin level. Helicobacter 2015; 20: 11–18. DOI: 10.1111/hel.12170.

[88] Azab SF, Esh AM. Serum hepcidin levels in *Helicobacter pylori*-infected children with iron-deficiency anemia: a case-control study. Ann Hematol. 2013; 92: 1477–1483. DOI: 10.1007/s00277-013-1813-2.

[89] Yip R, Limburg PJ, Ahlquist DA, Carpenter HA, O'Neill A, Kruse D, et al. Pervasive occult gastrointestinal bleeding in an Alaska native population with prevalent iron deficiency. Role of *Helicobacter pylori* gastritis. JAMA 1997; 277: 1135–1139.

[90] Kang JM, Kim N, Lee BH, Park HK, Jo HJ, Shin CM, et al. Risk factors for peptic ulcer bleeding in terms of *Helicobacter pylori*, NSAIDs, and antiplatelet agents. Scand J Gastroenterol. 2011; 46: 1295–1301. DOI: 10.3109/00365521.2011.605468.

[91] Musumba C, Jorgensen A, Sutton L, Van Eker D, Moorcroft J, Hopkins M, et al. The relative contribution of NSAIDs and *Helicobacter pylori* to the aetiology of endoscopically-diagnosed peptic ulcer disease: observations from a tertiary referral hospital in the UK between 2005 and 2010. Aliment Pharmacol Ther. 2012; 36: 48–56. DOI: 10.1111/j.1365-2036.2012.05118.x.

[92] Vergara M, Catalan M, Gisbert JP, Calvet X. Meta-analysis: role of *Helicobacter pylori* eradication in the prevention of peptic ulcer in NSAID users. Aliment Pharmacol Ther. 2005; 21: 1411–1418.

[93] De Leest HT, Steen KS, Bloemena E, Lems WF, Kuipers EJ, Van de Laar MA, et al. *Helicobacter pylori* eradication in patients on long-term treatment with NSAIDs reduces the severity of gastritis: a randomized controlled trial. J Clin Gastroenterol. 2009; 43: 140–146. DOI: 10.1097/MCG.0b013e3181595b40.

[94] Sokic-Milutinovic A, Krstic M, Rozer-Smolovic B, Alempijevic T. Role of *Helicobacter pylori* infection in gastroduodenal damage in patients starting NSAID therapy: 4 Months follow-up study. Dig Dis Sci. 2010; 55: 2887–2892. DOI: 10.1007/s10620-009-1097-5.

[95] Song HJ, Kwon JW, Kim N, Park YS. Cost effectiveness associated with *Helicobacter pylori* screening and eradication in patients taking nonsteroidal anti-inflammatory drugs and/or aspirin. Gut Liver. 2013; 7: 182–189. DOI: 10.5009/gnl.2013.7.2.182.

[96] Afifi MT, Abd El–Aziz HK, Hamed NA, Barghash NA, Abdo A, Gamal M. Role of *Helicobacter pylori* in refractory iron deficiency anaemia. Br J Biomed Sci. 2009; 66: 133–136.

[97] Boyanova L. Role of *Helicobacter pylori* virulence factors for iron acquisition from gastric epithelial cells of the host and impact on bacterial colonization. Future Microbiol. 2011; 6: 843–846. DOI: 10.2217/fmb.11.75.

[98] Ge R, Sun X. Iron trafficking system in *Helicobacter pylori*. Biometals 2012; 25: 247–258. DOI: 10.1007/s10534-011-9512-8.

[99] Davis RE. Clinical chemistry of vitamin B12. Adv Clin Chem. 1985; 24: 163–216.

[100] Herbert V. Staging vitamin B12 (cobalamin) status in vegetarians. Am J Clin Nutr. 1994; 59: 1213S–1222S.

[101] Andrés E, Loukili NH, Noel E, Kaltenbach G, Abdelgheni MB, Perrin AE, et al. Vitamin B12 (cobalamin) deficiency in elderly patients. CMAJ 2004; 171: 251–259.

[102] Dali-Youcef N, Andres E. An update on cobalamin deficiency in adults. QJM 2009; 102: 17–28. DOI: 10.1093/qjmed/hcn138.

[103] Carmel R, Johnson CS, Weiner JM. Pernicious anemia in Latin Americans is not a disease of the elderly. Arch Intern Med. 1987; 147: 1995–1996.

[104] Carmel R. Prevalence of undiagnosed pernicious anemia in the elderly. Arch Intern Med. 1996; 156: 1097–1100.

[105] Toh BH, van Driel IR, Gleeson PA. Pernicious anemia. N Engl J Med. 1997; 337: 1441–1448.

[106] Jimenez C, Bustos M, Besses C. The irreplaceable image: a patient with subacute degeneration of the spinal cord secondary to pernicious anemia. Haematologica 2001; 86: 444.

[107] Seshadri S, Beiser A, Selhub J, Jacques PF, Rosenberg IH, D'Agostino RB, et al. Plasma homocysteine as a risk factor for dementia and Alzheimer's disease. N Engl J Med. 2002; 346: 476–483.

[108] Hooshmand B, Solomon A, Kareholt I, Leiviska J, Rusanen M, Ahtiluoto S, et al. Homocysteine and holotranscobalamin and the risk of Alzheimer disease: a longitudinal study. Neurology 2010; 75: 1408–1414. DOI: 10.1212/WNL.0b013e3181f88162.

[109] Werder SF. Cobalamin deficiency, hyperhomocysteinemia, and dementia. Neuropsychiatr Dis Treat. 2010; 6: 159–195.

[110] Hooshmand B, Solomon A, Kareholt I, Rusanen M, Hanninen T, Leiviska J, et al. Associations between serum homocysteine, holotranscobalamin, folate and cognition in the elderly: a longitudinal study. J Intern Med. 2012; 271: 204–212. DOI: 10.1111/j.1365-2796.2011.02484.x.

[111] Tiemeier H, van Tuijl HR, Hofman A, Meijer J, Kiliaan AJ, Breteler MM. Vitamin B12, folate, and homocysteine in depression: the Rotterdam Study. Am J Psychiat. 2002; 159: 2099–2101.

[112] Kaptan K, Beyan C. Does hyperhomocysteinemia due to vitamin B12 deficiency associated with *Helicobacter pylori* infection has a role on cerebral stroke? Med Sci Monit. 2002; 8: LE52–LE53; author reply LE53.

[113] Moghaddasi M, Mamarabadi M, Mirzadeh S, Freydoonnejad AA, Razjouyan H. Homocysteine, vitamin B12 and folate levels in Iranian patients with ischemic stroke. Neurol Res. 2010; 32: 953–956. DOI: 10.1179/016164110X12644252260475.

[114] Caldera A, Mora J, Kotler M, Eiger G. Pulmonary embolism in a patient with pernicious anemia and hyperhomocysteinemia. Chest 2002; 122: 1487–1488.

[115] Andrés E, Kurtz JE. Pulmonary embolism in pernicious anemia and hyperhomocysteinemia. Chest 2003; 124: 1181.

[116] Whincup PH, Mendall MA, Perry IJ, Strachan DP. Hyperhomocysteinaemia, *Helicobacter pylori*, and coronary heart disease. Heart 1997; 78: 524.

[117] O'Connor HJ, Axon AT, Dixon MF. Campylobacter–like organisms unusual in type A (pernicious anaemia) gastritis. Lancet 1984; 2: 1091.

[118] Fong TL, Dooley CP, Dehesa M, Cohen H, Carmel R, Fitzgibbons PL, et al. *Helicobacter pylori* infection in pernicious anemia: a prospective controlled study. Gastroenterology 1991; 100: 328–332.

[119] Saito M, Mori A, Irie T, Tanaka M, Morioka M. *Helicobacter pylori* infection is not associated with pernicious anemia in Japan. Rinsho Ketsueki. 2008; 49: 1569–1571. DOI: JST.JSTAGE/rinketsu/49.1569 pii.

[120] Blaser MJ, Perez-Perez GI, Lindenbaum J, Schneidman D, Van Deventer G, Marin-Sorensen M, et al. Association of infection due to *Helicobacter pylori* with specific upper gastrointestinal pathology. Rev Infect Dis. 1991; 13 Suppl 8: S704–S708.

[121] Suter PM, Golner BB, Goldin BR, Morrow FD, Russell RM. Reversal of protein-bound vitamin B12 malabsorption with antibiotics in atrophic gastritis. Gastroenterology 1991; 101: 1039–1045.

[122] Valle J, Kekki M, Sipponen P, Ihamaki T, Siurala M. Long-term course and consequences of *Helicobacter pylori* gastritis. Results of a 32-year follow-up study. Scand J Gastroenterol. 1996; 31: 546–550.

[123] Claeys D, Faller G, Appelmelk BJ, Negrini R, Kirchner T. The gastric H+,K+-ATPase is a major autoantigen in chronic *Helicobacter pylori* gastritis with body mucosa atrophy. Gastroenterology 1998; 115: 340–347.

[124] Kokkola A, Kosunen TU, Puolakkainen P, Sipponen P, Harkonen M, Laxen F, et al. Spontaneous disappearance of *Helicobacter pylori* antibodies in patients with advanced atrophic corpus gastritis. Apmis 2003; 111: 619–624.

[125] Carmel R. Current concepts in cobalamin deficiency. Annu Rev Med. 2000; 51: 357–375. DOI: 10.1146/annurev.med.51.1.357.

[126] Kaptan K, Beyan C, Ural AU, Cetin T, Avcu F, Gulsen M, et al. *Helicobacter pylori*—is it a novel causative agent in Vitamin B12 deficiency? Arch Intern Med. 2000; 160: 1349–1353.

[127] Marino MC, de Oliveira CA, Rocha AM, Rocha GA, Clementino NC, Antunes LF, et al. Long-term effect of *Helicobacter pylori* eradication on plasma homocysteine in elderly patients with cobalamin deficiency. Gut. 2007; 56: 469–474.

[128] Lahner E, Persechino S, Annibale B. Micronutrients (other than iron) and *Helicobacter pylori* infection: a systematic review. Helicobacter 2012; 17: 1–15. DOI: 10.1111/j.1523-5378.2011.00892.x.

[129] Kaplan HS, Rigler LG. Pernicious anemia and susceptibility to gastric neoplasms. J Lab Clin Med. 1947; 32: 644–653.

[130] Zamcheck N, Grable E, Ley A, Norman L. Occurrence of gastric cancer among patients with pernicious anemia at the Boston City Hospital. N Engl J Med. 1955; 252: 1103–1110.

[131] Berkson J, Comfort MW, Butt HR. Occurrence of gastric cancer in persons with achlorhydria and eith pernicious anemia. Proc Staff Meet Mayo Clin. 1956; 31: 583–596.

[132] Payne RW. Pernicious anaemia and gastric cancer in England and Wales. Br Med J. 1961; 1: 1807–1809.

[133] Vannella L, Lahner E, Osborn J, Annibale B. Systematic review: gastric cancer incidence in pernicious anaemia. Aliment Pharmacol Ther. 2013; 37: 375–382. DOI: 10.1111/apt.12177.

[134] Carmel R. Megaloblastic anemias: disorders of impaired DNA synthesis. In: Greer JP, Arber DA, Glader B, List AF, Means RTJ, Paraskevas F, et al., editors. Wintrobe's Clinical Hematology. 13 Ed. Philadelphia, PA: Lippincott Williams & Wilkins; 2013. p. 927–953.

[135] Liel MS, Carverley DC. Thrombopcytopenia caused by immunologic platelet destruction In: Greer JP, Arber DA, Glader B, List AF, Means RTJ, Paraskevas F, et al., editors. Wintrobe's Clinical Hematology. 13 Ed. Philadelphia, PA: Lippincott Williams & Wilkins; 2013. p. 1061–1076.

[136] Frederiksen H, Schmidt K. The incidence of idiopathic thrombocytopenic purpura in adults increases with age. Blood 1999; 94: 909–913.

[137] Neunert C, Lim W, Crowther M, Cohen A, Solberg L, Jr., Crowther MA. The American Society of Hematology 2011 evidence-based practice guideline for immune thrombocytopenia. Blood 2011; 117: 4190–4207. DOI: 10.1182/blood-2010-08-302984.

[138] Pizzuto J, Ambriz R. Therapeutic experience on 934 adults with idiopathic thrombocytopenic purpura: Multicentric Trial of the Cooperative Latin American group on Hemostasis and Thrombosis. Blood 1984; 64: 1179–1183.

[139] Rodeghiero F, Stasi R, Gernsheimer T, Michel M, Provan D, Arnold DM, et al. Standardization of terminology, definitions and outcome criteria in immune thrombocytopenic purpura of adults and children: report from an international working group. Blood 2009; 113: 2386–2393. DOI: 10.1182/blood-2008-07-162503.

[140] British Society for Haematology. Guidelines for the investigation and management of idiopathic thrombocytopenic purpura in adults, children and in pregnancy. Br J Haematol. 2003; 120: 574–596.

[141] García-Pérez A, Valverde de La Osa J, Giménez Samper M, Alonso García I. Resolution of an autoimmune thrombocytopenic purpura after eradicating treatment of *Helicobacter pylori*. Sangre (Barc). 1999; 44: 387–388.

[142] Tohda S, Ohkusa T. Resolution of refractory idiopathic thrombocytopenic purpura after eradication of *Helicobacter pylori*. Am J Hematol. 2000; 65: 329–330.

[143] Goto H, Kikuta T, Ota A, Tsuji H, Hino R. Successful treatment of refractory idiopathic thrombocytopenic purpura by eradication of *Helicobacter pylori*. Rinsho Ketsueki. 2001; 42: 1192–1194.

[144] Mukai M, Kon Y, Notoya A, Kohno M. *Helicobacter pylori* associated with idiopathic thrombocytopenic purpura. Am J Med. 2002; 113: 169–171.

[145] Asaumi N, Niiya K, Shibakura M, Yoshida C, Niiya M, Tanimoto M. Secondary eradication of *Helicobacter pylori* was effective against refractory idiopathic thrombocytopenic purpura. Blood Coagul Fibrinolysis. 2003; 14: 785–786.

[146] Takechi T, Unemoto J, Ishihara M, Hosokawa T, Zushi N, Shiraishi T, et al. Idiopathic thrombocytopenic purpura associated with *Helicobacter pylori* infection. Pediatr Int. 2006; 48: 76–78.

[147] Grimaz S, Damiani D, Brosolo P, Skert C, Geromin A, de Pretis G. Resolution of thrombocytopenia after treatment for *Helicobacter pylori*: a case report. Haematologica 1999; 84: 283–284.

[148] Soldinger E, Pilia MC, Piubello W, Nadali G. Multi-resistant idiopathic thrombocytopenia successfully treated by eradication of *Helicobacter pylori*. Dig Liver Dis. 2001; 33: 732.

[149] Candelli M, Nista EC, Pignataro G, Gasbarrini G, Gasbarrini A. Idiopathic thrombocytopenic purpura and *Helicobacter pylori* infection. Scand J Gastroenterol. 2003; 38: 569–570.

[150] Kurekci AE, Atay AA, Sarici SU, Ozcan O. Complete platelet recovery after treatment of *Helicobacter pylori* infection in a child with chronic immune thrombocytopenic purpura: a case report. Pediatr Hematol Oncol. 2004; 21: 593–596.

[151] Gasbarrini A, Franceschi F, Tartaglione R, Landolfi R, Pola P, Gasbarrini G. Regression of autoimmune thrombocytopenia after eradication of *Helicobacter pylori*. Lancet 1998; 352: 878.

[152] Emilia G, Longo G, Luppi M, Gandini G, Morselli M, Ferrara L, et al. *Helicobacter pylori* eradication can induce platelet recovery in idiopathic thrombocytopenic purpura. Blood 2001; 97: 812–814.

[153] Emilia G, Luppi M, Morselli M, Potenza L, D'Apollo N, Torelli G. *Helicobacter pylori* infection and idiopathic thrombocytopenic purpura. Br J Haematol. 2002; 118: 1198–1199.

[154] Veneri D, Franchini M, Gottardi M, D'Adda M, Ambrosetti A, Krampera M, et al. Efficacy of *Helicobacter pylori* eradication in raising platelet count in adult patients with idiopathic thrombocytopenic purpura. Haematologica 2002; 87: 1177–1179.

[155] Veneri D, Franchini M. Onset of Idiopathic Thrombocythemia after *Helicobacter pylori* Eradication. Helicobacter 2005; 10: 95.

[156] Stasi R, Rossi Z, Stipa E, Amadori S, Newland AC, Provan D. *Helicobacter pylori* eradication in the management of patients with idiopathic thrombocytopenic purpura. Am J Med. 2005; 118: 414–419.

[157] Emilia G, Luppi M, Zucchini P, Morselli M, Potenza L, Forghieri F, et al. *Helicobacter pylori* infection and chronic immune thrombocytopenic purpura: long–term results of bacterium eradication and association with bacterium virulence profiles. Blood 2007; 110: 3833–3841. DOI: 10.1182/blood-2006-12-063222.

[158] Scandellari R, Allemand E, Vettore S, Plebani M, Randi ML, Fabris F. Platelet response to *Helicobacter pylori* eradication therapy in adult chronic idiopathic thrombocytopenic purpura seems to be related to the presence of anticytotoxin-associated gene A antibodies. Blood Coagul Fibrinolysis. 2009; 20: 108–113. DOI: 10.1097/MBC.0b013e32832315d8.

[159] Sayan O, Akyol Erikci A, Ozturk A. The Efficacy of *Helicobacter pylori* eradication in the treatment of idiopathic thrombocytopenic purpura—the first study in Turkey. Acta Haematol. 2006; 116: 146–149. DOI: 10.1159/000093648.

[160] Suvajdzic N, Stankovic B, Artiko V, Cvejic T, Bulat V, Bakrac M, et al. *Helicobacter pylori* eradication can induce platelet recovery in chronic idiopathic thrombocytopenic purpura. Platelets 2006; 17: 227–230.

[161] Kohda K, Kuga T, Kogawa K, Kanisawa Y, Koike K, Kuroiwa G, et al. Effect of *Helicobacter pylori* eradication on platelet recovery in Japanese patients with chronic idiopathic thrombocytopenic purpura and secondary autoimmune thrombocytopenic purpura. Br J Haematol. 2002; 118: 584–588.

[162] Kohda K, Niitsu Y. *Helicobacter pylori* infection and idiopathic thrombocytopenic purpura. Nippon Rinsho. 2003; 61: 644–649.

[163] Ando K, Shimamoto T, Tauchi T, Ito Y, Kuriyama Y, Gotoh A, et al. Can eradication therapy for *Helicobacter pylori* really improve the thrombocytopenia in idiopathic thrombocytopenic purpura? Our experience and a literature review. Int J Hematol. 2003; 77: 239–244.

[164] Hashino S, Mori A, Suzuki S, Izumiyama K, Kahata K, Yonezumi M, et al. Platelet recovery in patients with idiopathic thrombocytopenic purpura after eradication of *Helicobacter pylori*. Int J Hematol. 2003; 77: 188–191.

[165] Hino M, Yamane T, Park K, Takubo T, Ohta K, Kitagawa S, et al. Platelet recovery after eradication of *Helicobacter pylori* in patients with idiopathic thrombocytopenic purpura. Ann Hematol. 2003; 82: 30–32.

[166] Kato A, Kato H, Hirashima N, Sakamoto T, Nukaya H, Ito K, et al. Evaluation of the efficacy of an *Helicobacter pylori* eradication treatment for idiopathic thrombocytopenic purpura patients. Nippon Shokakibyo Gakkai Zasshi. 2004; 101: 1209–1216.

[167] Ando T, Tsuzuki T, Mizuno T, Minami M, Ina K, Kusugami K, et al. Characteristics of *Helicobacter pylori*-induced gastritis and the effect of *H. pylori* eradication in pa-

tients with chronic idiopathic thrombocytopenic purpura. Helicobacter 2004; 9: 443–452.

[168] Nomura S, Inami N, Kanazawa S. The effects of *Helicobacter pylori* eradication on chemokine production in patients with immune thrombocytopenic purpura. Eur J Haematol. 2004; 72: 304–305.

[169] Sato R, Murakami K, Watanabe K, Okimoto T, Miyajima H, Ogata M, et al. Effect of *Helicobacter pylori* eradication on platelet recovery in patients with chronic idiopathic thrombocytopenic purpura. Arch Intern Med. 2004; 164: 1904–1907.

[170] Takahashi T, Yujiri T, Shinohara K, Inoue Y, Sato Y, Fujii Y, et al. Molecular mimicry by *Helicobacter pylori* CagA protein may be involved in the pathogenesis of *H. pylori*-associated chronic idiopathic thrombocytopenic purpura. Br J Haematol. 2004; 124: 91–96.

[171] Fujimura K. *Helicobacter pylori* infection and idiopathic thrombocytopenic purpura. Int J Hematol. 2005; 81: 113–118.

[172] Inaba T, Mizuno M, Take S, Suwaki K, Honda T, Kawai K, et al. Eradication of *Helicobacter pylori* increases platelet count in patients with idiopathic thrombocytopenic purpura in Japan. Eur J Clin Invest. 2005; 35: 214–219.

[173] Tsutsumi Y, Kanamori H, Yamato H, Ehira N, Kawamura T, Umehara S, et al. Randomized study of *Helicobacter pylori* eradication therapy and proton pump inhibitor monotherapy for idiopathic thrombocytopenic purpura. Ann Hematol. 2005; 84: 807–811.

[174] Suzuki T, Matsushima M, Masui A, Watanabe K, Takagi A, Ogawa Y, et al. Effect of *Helicobacter pylori* eradication in patients with chronic idiopathic thrombocytopenic purpura–a randomized controlled trial. Am J Gastroenterol. 2005; 100: 1265–1270.

[175] Asahi A, Kuwana M, Suzuki H, Hibi T, Kawakami Y, Ikeda Y. Effects of a *Helicobacter pylori* eradication regimen on anti-platelet autoantibody response in infected and uninfected patients with idiopathic thrombocytopenic purpura. Haematologica 2006; 91: 1436–1437.

[176] Ishiyama M, Teramura M, Iwabe K, Kato T, Motoji T. Clonally expanded T-cells in the peripheral blood of patients with idiopathic thrombocytopenic purpura and *Helicobacter pylori* infection. Int J Hematol. 2006; 83: 147–151.

[177] Satake M, Nishikawa J, Fukagawa Y, Akashi K, Okamoto T, Yoshida T, et al. The long-term efficacy of *Helicobacter pylori* eradication therapy in patients with idiopathic thrombocytopenic purpura. J Gastroenterol Hepatol. 2007; 22: 2233–2237. DOI: 10.1111/j.1440-1746.2007.04845.x.

[178] Kodama M, Kitadai Y, Ito M, Kai H, Masuda H, Tanaka S, et al. Immune Response to CagA protein is associated with improved platelet count after *Helicobacter pylori* erad-

ication in patients with idiopathic thrombocytopenic purpura. Helicobacter 2007; 12: 36–42.

[179] Asahi A, Nishimoto T, Okazaki Y, Suzuki H, Masaoka T, Kawakami Y, et al. *Helicobacter pylori* eradication shifts monocyte Fcgamma receptor balance toward inhibitory FcgammaRIIB in immune thrombocytopenic purpura patients. J Clin Invest. 2008; 118: 2939–2949. DOI: 10.1172/JCI34496.

[180] Suzuki T, Matsushima M, Shirakura K, Koike J, Masui A, Takagi A, et al. Association of inflammatory cytokine gene polymorphisms with platelet recovery in idiopathic thrombocytopenic purpura patients after the eradication of *Helicobacter pylori*. Digestion 2008; 77: 73–78. DOI: 10.1159/000121392.

[181] Tsumoto C, Tominaga K, Okazaki H, Tanigawa T, Yamagami H, Watanabe K, et al. Long-term efficacy of *Helicobacter pylori* eradication in patients with idiopathic thrombocytopenic purpura: 7-year follow-up prospective study. Ann Hematol. 2009; 88: 789–793. DOI: 10.1007/s00277-008-0667-5.

[182] Sato R, Murakami K, Okimoto T, Watanabe K, Kodama M, Fujioka T. Development of corpus atrophic gastritis may be associated with *Helicobacter pylori*-related idiopathic thrombocytopenic purpura. J Gastroenterol. 2011; 46: 991–997. DOI: 10.1007/s00535-011-0416-8.

[183] Kikuchi T, Kobayashi T, Yamashita T, Ohashi K, Sakamaki H, Akiyama H. Eight-year follow-up of patients with immune thrombocytopenic purpura related to *H. pylori* infection. Platelets 2011; 22: 59–62. DOI: 10.3109/09537104.2010.515272.

[184] Kong R, Qiu HC, Wu PF, Niu XH, Shen WX, Wang Y. Clinical significance of *Helicobacter pylori* in pathogenesis of idiopathic thrombocytopenic purpura. Zhongguo Shi Yan Xue Ye Xue Za Zhi. 2008; 16: 1222–1226. DOI: 1009-2137(2008)05-1222-05 pii.

[185] Wu S, Li Y, Jian Z, Tang F. Anti-*Helicobacter pylori* treatment in patients with idiopathic thrombocytopenic purpura. Zhong Nan Da Xue Xue Bao Yi Xue Ban. 2009; 34: 1251–1254.

[186] Rostami N, Keshtkar-Jahromi M, Rahnavardi M, Esfahani FS. Effect of eradication of *Helicobacter pylori* on platelet recovery in patients with chronic idiopathic thrombocytopenic purpura: a controlled trial. Am J Hematol. 2008; 83: 376–381. DOI: 10.1002/ajh.21125.

[187] Payandeh M, Sohrabi N, Zare ME, Kansestani AN, Hashemian AH. Platelet count response to *Helicobacter pylori* eradication in Iranian patients with idiopathic thrombocytopenic purpura. Mediterr J Hematol Infect Dis. 2012; 4: e2012056. DOI: 10.4084/MJHID.2012.056.

[188] Tag HS, Lee HS, Jung SH, Kim BK, Kim SB, Lee A, et al. Effects of *Helicobacter pylori* eradication in patients with immune thrombocytopenic purpura. Korean J Hematol. 2010; 45: 127–132. DOI: 10.5045/kjh.2010.45.2.127.

[189] Campuzano-Maya G. Proof of an association between *Helicobacter pylori* and idiopathic thrombocytopenic purpura in Latin America. Helicobacter 2007; 12: 265–273. DOI: 10.1111/j.1523-5378.2007.00502.x.

[190] Jackson SC, Beck P, Buret AG, O'Connor PM, Meddings J, Pineo G, et al. Long term platelet responses to *Helicobacter pylori* eradication in Canadian patients with immune thrombocytopenic purpura. Int J Hematol. 2008; 88: 212–218. DOI: 10.1007/s12185-008-0138-8.

[191] Campuzano-Maya G. Hematologic manifestations of *Helicobacter pylori* infection. World J Gastroenterol. 2014; 20: 12818–12838. DOI: 10.3748/wjg.v20.i36.12818.

[192] Jarque I, Andreu R, Llopis I, De la Rubia J, Gomis F, Senent L, et al. Absence of platelet response after eradication of *Helicobacter pylori* infection in patients with chronic idiopathic thrombocytopenic purpura. Br J Haematol. 2001; 115: 1002–1003.

[193] Michel M, Khellaf M, Desforges L, Lee K, Schaeffer A, Godeau B, et al. Autoimmune thrombocytopenic purpura and *Helicobacter pylori* infection. Arch Intern Med. 2002; 162: 1033–1036.

[194] Ahn ER, Tiede MP, Jy W, Bidot CJ, Fontana V, Ahn YS. Platelet activation in *Helicobacter pylori*-associated idiopathic thrombocytopenic purpura: eradication reduces platelet activation but seldom improves platelet counts. Acta Haematol. 2006; 116: 19–24.

[195] Estrada-Gomez RA, Parra-Ortega I, Martinez-Barreda C, Ruiz-Arguelles GJ. *Helicobacter pylori* infection and thrombocytopenia: a single-institution experience in Mexico. Rev Invest Clin. 2007; 59: 112–115.

[196] Jaing TH, Yang CP, Hung IJ, Chiu CH, Chang KW. Efficacy of *Helicobacter pylori* eradication on platelet recovery in children with chronic idiopathic thrombocytopenic purpura. Acta Paediatr. 2003; 92: 1153–1157.

[197] Hayashi H, Okuda M, Aoyagi N, Yoshiyama M, Miyashiro E, Kounami S, et al. *Helicobacter pylori* infection in children with chronic idiopathic thrombocytopenic purpura. Pediatr Int. 2005; 47: 292–295.

[198] Hamidieh AA, Arzanian MT, Gachkar L, Pasha F. *Helicobacter pylori* infection in children with chronic idiopathic thrombocytopenic purpura. J Pediatr Hematol Oncol. 2008; 30: 96–97. DOI: 10.1097/MPH.0b013e3181615600.

[199] Rajantie J, Klemola T. *Helicobacter pylori* and idiopathic thrombocytopenic purpura in children. Blood 2003; 101: 1660.

[200] Neefjes VM, Heijboer H, Tamminga RY. *H. pylori* infection in childhood chronic immune thrombocytopenic purpura. Haematologica 2007; 92: 576.

[201] Ferrara M, Capozzi L, Russo R. Influence of *Helicobacter pylori* infection associated with iron deficiency anaemia on growth in pre-adolescent children. Hematology 2009; 14: 173–176. DOI: 10.1179/102453309X402287.

[202] Russo G, Miraglia V, Branciforte F, Matarese SM, Zecca M, Bisogno G, et al. Effect of eradication of *Helicobacter pylori* in children with chronic immune thrombocytopenia: a prospective, controlled, multicenter study. Pediatr Blood Cancer. 2011; 56: 273–278. DOI: 10.1002/pbc.22770.

[203] Yetgin S, Demir H, Arslan D, Unal S, Kocak N. Autoimmune thrombocytopenic purpura and *Helicobacter pylori* infection effectivity during childhood. Am J Hematol. 2005; 78: 318.

[204] Loffredo G, Marzano MG, Migliorati R, Miele E, Menna F, Poggi V, et al. The relationship between immune thrombocytopenic purpura and *Helicobacter pylori* infection in children: where is the truth? Eur J Pediatr. 2007; 166: 1067–1068.

[205] Bisogno G, Errigo G, Rossetti F, Sainati L, Pusiol A, Da Dalt L, et al. The role of *Helicobacter pylori* in children with chronic idiopathic thrombocytopenic purpura. J Pediatr Hematol Oncol. 2008; 30: 53–57. DOI: 10.1097/MPH.0b013e3181615613.

[206] Teawtrakul N, Sawadpanich K, Sirijerachai C, Chansung K, Wanitpongpun C. Clinical characteristics and treatment outcomes in patients with *Helicobacter pylori*-positive chronic immune thrombocytopenic purpura. Platelets 2014; 25: 548–551. DOI: 10.3109/09537104.2013.841883.

[207] Treepongkaruna S, Sirachainan N, Kanjanapongkul S, Winaichatsak A, Sirithorn S, Sumritsopak R, et al. Absence of platelet recovery following *Helicobacter pylori* eradication in childhood chronic idiopathic thrombocytopenic purpura: a multi-center randomized controlled trial. Pediatr Blood Cancer. 2009; 53: 72–77. DOI: 10.1002/pbc.21991.

[208] Veres G, Karoczkai I, Bodanszky H, Marosi A, Magyarossi E, Dezsofi A, et al. The role of *Helicobacter pylori* infection in children with chronic immune thrombocytopenic purpura. Orv Hetil. 2009; 150: 801–804. DOI: 10.1556/OH.2009.28581.

[209] Provan D, Stasi R, Newland AC, Blanchette VS, Bolton-Maggs P, Bussel JB, et al. International consensus report on the investigation and management of primary immune thrombocytopenia. Blood 2010; 115: 168–186. DOI: 10.1182/blood-2009-06-225565.

[210] Bai Y, Wang Z, Bai X, Yu Z, Cao L, Zhang W, et al. Cross-reaction of antibody against *Helicobacter pylori* urease B with platelet glycoprotein IIIa and its significance in the pathogenesis of immune thrombocytopenic purpura. Int J Hematol. 2009; 89: 142–149. DOI: 10.1007/s12185-008-0247-4.

[211] Franchini M, Cruciani M, Mengoli C, Pizzolo G, Veneri D. Effect of *Helicobacter pylori* eradication on platelet count in idiopathic thrombocytopenic purpura: a systematic review and meta-analysis. J Antimicrob Chemother. 2007; 60: 237–246.

[212] Stasi R, Sarpatwari A, Segal JB, Osborn J, Evangelista ML, Cooper N, et al. Effects of eradication of *Helicobacter pylori* infection in patients with immune thrombocytopenic purpura: a systematic review. Blood 2009; 113: 1231–1240. DOI: 10.1182/blood-2008-07-167155.

[213] Arnold DM, Bernotas A, Nazi I, Stasi R, Kuwana M, Liu Y, et al. Platelet count response to *H. pylori* treatment in patients with immune thrombocytopenic purpura with and without *H. pylori* infection: a systematic review. Haematologica 2009; 94: 850–856. DOI: 10.3324/haematol.2008.005348.

[214] Gupta V, Eden AJ, Mills MJ. *Helicobacter pylori* and autoimmune neutropenia. Clin Lab Haematol. 2002; 24: 183–185.

[215] Papadaki HA, Pontikoglou C, Stavroulaki E, Minadakis G, Eliopoulos DA, Pyrovolaki K, et al. High prevalence of *Helicobacter pylori* infection and monoclonal gammopathy of undetermined significance in patients with chronic idiopathic neutropenia. Ann Hematol. 2005; 84: 317–320.

[216] Papadaki HA, Pontikoglou C, Eliopoulos DG, Pyrovolaki K, Spyridaki R, Eliopoulos GD. *Helicobacter pylori* infection is probably the cause of chronic idiopathic neutropenia (CIN)-associated splenomegaly. Am J Hematol. 2006; 81: 142–144.

[217] Lim W, Crowther MA, Eikelboom JW. Management of antiphospholipid antibody syndrome: a systematic review. JAMA 2006; 295: 1050–1057. DOI: 10.1001/jama.295.9.1050.

[218] Cicconi V, Carloni E, Franceschi F, Nocente R, Silveri NG, Manna R, et al. Disappearance of antiphospholipid antibodies syndrome after *Helicobacter pylori* eradication. Am J Med. 2001; 111: 163–164.

[219] Stasi R, Stipa E, Masi M, Oliva F, Sciarra A, Perrotti A, et al. Prevalence and clinical significance of elevated antiphospholipid antibodies in patients with idiopathic thrombocytopenic purpura. Blood 1994; 84: 4203–4208.

[220] Lipp E, von Felten A, Sax H, Muller D, Berchtold P. Antibodies against platelet glycoproteins and antiphospholipid antibodies in autoimmune thrombocytopenia. Eur J Haematol. 1998; 60: 283–288.

[221] Macchi L, Rispal P, Clofent-Sanchez G, Pellegrin JL, Nurden P, Leng B, et al. Antiplatelet antibodies in patients with systemic lupus erythematosus and the primary antiphospholipid antibody syndrome: their relationship with the observed thrombocytopenia. Br J Haematol. 1997; 98: 336–341.

[222] Costen MT, Parkin BT, Davison CR, Crick MP. Central serous chorioretinopathy and antiphospholipid antibodies-results of a pilot study. Eye 2004; 18: 938.

[223] Cotticelli L, Borrelli M, D'Alessio AC, Menzione M, Villani A, Piccolo G, et al. Central serous chorioretinopathy and *Helicobacter pylori*. Eur J Ophthalmol. 2006; 16: 274–278.

[224] Gok F, Ugur Y, Ozen S, Dagdeviren A. Pathogenesis-related adhesion molecules in Henoch–Schönlein vasculitis. Rheumatol Int. 2008; 28: 313–316. DOI: 10.1007/s00296-007-0437-z.

[225] Reinauer S, Megahed M, Goerz G, Ruzicka T, Borchard F, Susanto F, et al. Schönlein–Henoch purpura associated with gastric *Helicobacter pylori* infection. J Am Acad Dermatol. 1995; 33: 876–879.

[226] Cecchi R, Torelli E. Schönlein–Henoch purpura in association with duodenal ulcer and gastric *Helicobacter pylori* infection. J Dermatol. 1998; 25: 482–484.

[227] Novak J, Szekanecz Z, Sebesi J, Takats A, Demeter P, Bene L, et al. Elevated levels of anti-*Helicobacter pylori* antibodies in Henoch–Schönlein purpura. Autoimmunity. 2003; 36: 307–311.

[228] Fu KI, Yagi S, Mashimo Y, Sugitani K, Imamaki K, Yanagisawa M, et al. Regression of *Helicobacter pylori*-negative duodenal ulcers complicated by Schönlein–Henoch purpura with *H. pylori* eradication therapy: the first report. Dig Dis Sci. 2005; 50: 381–384.

[229] Mytinger JR, Patterson JW, Thibault ES, Webb J, Saulsbury FT. Henoch–Schönlein purpura associated with *Helicobacter pylori* infection in a child. Pediatr Dermatol. 2008; 25: 630–632. DOI: 10.1111/j.1525-1470.2008.00786.x.

[230] Grivceva-Panovska V, Grivceva Stardelova K, Serafimoski V. Henoch–Schönlein purpura in an adult patient: extragastric, cutaneous manifestation of *Helicobacter pylori* infection. Prilozi 2008; 29: 291–301.

[231] Hoshino C. Adult onset Schönlein–Henoch purpura associated with *Helicobacter pylori* infection. Intern Med. 2009; 48: 847–851. DOI: JST.JSTAGE/internalmedicine/48.1718 pii.

[232] Mozrzymas R, d'Amore ES, Montini G, Guariso G. Schönlein–Henoch vasculitis and chronic *Helicobacter pylori* associated gastritis and duodenal ulcer: a case report. Pediatr Med Chir. 1997; 19: 467–468.

[233] Shin JI, Koh H, Lee JS. Henoch–Schönlein purpura associated with *Helicobacter pylori* infection: the pathogenic roles of IgA, C3, and cryoglobulins? Pediatr Dermatol. 2009; 26: 768–769. DOI: 10.1111/j.1525-1470.2009.01039.x.

[234] International Myeloma Working Group. Criteria for the classification of monoclonal gammopathies, multiple myeloma and related disorders: a report of the International Myeloma Working Group. Br J Haematol. 2003; 121: 749–757.

[235] Osler W, McRae T, editors. Diseases of the stomach. The principles and practice of medicine. New York: Appleton; 1920. p. 425.

[236] Twomey JJ, Laughter AH, Villanueva ND, Kao YS, Lidsky MD, Jordan PH, Jr. Gastric secretory and serologic studies on patients with neoplastic and immunologic disorders. Arch Intern Med. 1971; 128: 746–749.

[237] Doberauer C, Sanner B, Henning B. Multiple myeloma involving the stomach with vitamin B12 deficiency. Eur J Gastroenterol Hepatol. 1999; 11: 205–207.

[238] Chanarin I. The megaloblastic aenemias. 2 Ed. Oxford: Blackell Scientific Pubications; 1979.

[239] Elsborg L, Mosbech J. Pernicious anaemia as a risk factor in gastric cancer. Acta Med Scand. 1979; 206: 315–318.

[240] Borch K. Epidemiologic, clinicopathologic, and economic aspects of gastroscopic screening of patients with pernicious anemia. Scand J Gastroenterol. 1986; 21: 21–30.

[241] Hsing AW, Hansson LE, McLaughlin JK, Nyren O, Blot WJ, Ekbom A, et al. Pernicious anemia and subsequent cancer. A population-based cohort study. Cancer 1993; 71: 745–750.

[242] Carmel R. Megaloblastic anemias: disorders of impaired DNA synthesis. In: Greer JP, Foerster J, Lukens J, Rodgers GM, Paraskevas F, Glader G, editors. Wintrobe's Clinical Hematology. 10 Ed. Philadelphia, PA: Lippincott Williams & Wilkins; 2004. p. 1367–1395.

[243] González-Cueto D, Bruno S, Bustos-Fernández LM, Narbaitz M. Gastric solitary plasmacytoma associated with *Helicobacter pylori* infection. Acta Gastroenterol Latinoam. 1999; 29: 119–123.

[244] Kato K, Sugitani M, Nagata T, Nishinarita S, Kawamura F, Takahashi Y, et al. A case of gastric plasmacytoma associated with *Helicobacter pylori* infection: improvement of abnormal endoscopic and EUS findings after *H. pylori* eradication. Gastrointest Endosc. 2001; 53: 352–355.

[245] Papadaki HA, Skordilis P, Minadakis G, Roussomoustakaki M, Katrinakis G, Psyllaki M, et al. Complete regression of primary gastric plasmacytoma following *Helicobacter pylori* eradication. Ann Hematol. 2003; 82: 589–592.

[246] Tursi A, Modeo ME. Monoclonal gammopathy of undetermined significance predisposing to *Helicobacter pylori*-related gastric mucosa-associated lymphoid tissue lymphoma. J Clin Gastroenterol. 2002; 34: 147–149.

[247] Braggio E, Fonseca R. Genomic abnormalities of Waldenström macroglobulinemia and related low-grade B-cell lymphomas. Clin Lymphoma Myeloma Leuk. 2013; 13: 198–201. DOI: 10.1016/j.clml.2013.02.015.

[248] Feingold ML, Goldstein MJ, Lieberman PH. Multiple myeloma involving the stomach. Report of a case with gastroscopic observations. Gastrointest Endosc. 1969; 16: 107–110.

[249] Kyle RA, Pierre RV, Bayrd ED. Multiple myeloma and acute myelomonocytic leukemia. N Engl J Med. 1970; 283: 1121–1125.

[250] Law IP, Blom J. Second malignancies in patients with multiple myeloma. Oncology 1977; 34: 20–24.

[251] Bergsagel DE, Bailey AJ, Langley GR, MacDonald RN, White DF, Miller AB. The chemotherapy on plasma-cell myeloma and the incidence of acute leukemia. N Engl J Med. 1979; 301: 743–748.

[252] Nelson RS. Tumores malignos del estómago distintos del carcinoma. In: Berk JE, Haubrich WS, Kalser M, Roth JLA, Vilardell F, editors. Gastroenterología. Henry Bockus. 3th Ed. Barcelona, España: Salvat Editores, S.A. ; 1980. p. 1058–1078.

[253] Brouet JC, Fermand JP, Laurent G, Grange MJ, Chevalier A, Jacquillat C, et al. The association of chronic lymphocytic leukaemia and multiple myeloma: a study of eleven patients. Br J Haematol. 1985; 59: 55–66.

[254] Kaufmann H, Ackermann J, Nosslinger T, Kromer E, Zojer N, Schreiber S, et al. Absence of clonal chromosomal relationship between concomitant B-CLL and multiple myeloma—a report on two cases. Ann Hematol. 2001; 80: 474–478.

[255] Wöhrer S, Isaacson PG, Raderer M. Complete regression of primary gastric plasmacytoma following *Helicobacter pylori* eradication. Ann Hematol. 2004; 83: 666.

[256] Wöhrer S, Raderer M, Streubel B, Chott A, Drach J. Concomitant occurrence of MALT lymphoma and multiple myeloma. Ann Hematol. 2004; 83: 600–603.

[257] Malik AA, Ganti AK, Potti A, Levitt R, Hanley JF. Role of *Helicobacter pylori* infection in the incidence and clinical course of monoclonal gammopathy of undetermined significance. Am J Gastroenterol. 2002; 97: 1371–1374.

[258] Wolkersdorfer GW, Haase M, Morgner A, Baretton G, Miehlke S. Monoclonal gammopathy of undetermined significance and russell body formation in *Helicobacter pylori* gastritis. Helicobacter 2006; 11: 506–510.

[259] Rajkumar SV, Kyle RA, Plevak MF, Murray JA, Therneau TM. *Helicobacter pylori* infection and monoclonal gammopathy of undetermined significance. Br J Haematol. 2002; 119: 706–708.

[260] Lehtinen M, Ogmundsdottir HM, Bloigu A, Hakulinen T, Hemminki E, Gudnadottir M, et al. Associations between three types of maternal bacterial infection and risk of leukemia in the offspring. Am J Epidemiol. 2005; 162: 662–667. DOI: 10.1093/aje/kwi261.

[261] Diamantidis MD, Ioannidou-Papagiannaki E, Kountouras J, Mandala E, Tsapournas G, Frida-Michailidou I, et al. High prevalence of *Helicobacter pylori* infection in Greek

patients with myelodysplastic syndromes. Acta Haematol. 2010; 124: 141–149. DOI: 10.1159/000319629.

[262] Kawamata T, Tojo A. *Helicobacter pylori*-induced thrombocytosis clinically indistinguishable from essential thrombocythemia. Leuk Lymphoma. 2012; 53: 1423–1424. DOI: 10.3109/10428194.2011.653787.

[263] Fioredda F, Haupt R, Castagnola E, Barabino A, Micalizzi C, Dini G, et al. *Helicobacter pylori*-associated large gastric ulcer during treatment for childhood leukemia. J Pediatr Hematol Oncol. 2002; 24: 759–762.

[264] Dolatkhah R, Khoshbaten M, Asvadi Kermani I, Reza Bonyadi M, Ghojazadeh M, Sanaat Z, et al. Upper gastrointestinal bleedings in patients with hereditary coagulation disorders in Northwest of Iran: prevalence of *Helicobacter pylori* infection. Eur J Gastroenterol Hepatol. 2011; 23: 1172–1177. DOI: 10.1097/MEG.0b013e32834b0e7a.

[265] Schulman S, Rehnberg AS, Hein M, Hegedus O, Lindmarker P, Hellstrom PM. *Helicobacter pylori* causes gastrointestinal hemorrhage in patients with congenital bleeding disorders. Thromb Haemost. 2003; 89: 741–746.

[266] Braden B, Wenke A, Karich HJ, Dietrich CF, Scharrer I, Caspary WF, et al. Risk of gastrointestinal bleeding associated with Helicobacter pylori infection in patients with hemophilia or von Willebrand's syndrome. Helicobacter 1998; 3: 184–187.

[267] Tincani E, Bertoni G, Silingardi M, Ghirarduzzi A, Bedogni G, Iori I. Helicobacter pylori, a frequent and potentially dangerous guest in the gastroduodenal mucosa of anticoagulated patients. Am J Med. 2000; 108: 165–167.

Chapter 4

# Hematological Extradigestive Manifestations of *Helicobacter pylori* Infection in Childhood

Natalina Miguel

Additional information is available at the end of the chapter

http://dx.doi.org/10.5772/63827

**Abstract**

*Helicobacter pylori* infects more than 50% of the world population and is acquired in infancy. Higher prevalence is found in developing countries, and within geographic areas the predominance correlates inversely with socioeconomic status, especially with living conditions during childhood. Initially, in adults, *H. pylori* was only associated with gastric diseases, such as peptic ulcer, gastritis, gastric adenocarcinoma, and gastric mucosa-associated lymphoid tissue (MALT) lymphoma, and in childhood, with chronic gastritis and duodenal ulcers in children. Recently, *H. pylori* has been related to non-gastric diseases, including hematological disorders such as iron deficiency anemia (IDA), chronic idiopathic thrombocytopenia (cITP), and vitamin B12 deficiency. *H. pylori* can trigger autoimmune atrophic gastritis and be responsible initially for an oral iron refractory anemia. Other hematological associations have been made, such as an increased risk of childhood leukemia in children of *H. pylori*-infected mothers and gastric bleeding in children with coagulation pathologies. *H. pylori* infection is important in the immune pathogenesis of chronic gastric inflammation and hematological diseases. The diagnostic methodology is based on non-invasive (serology, C-urea breath test, stool HP antigen) and invasive tests. The scientific community discussed and incorporated in international consensus for the investigation and management of these hematological extragastric pathologies (IDA, cITP, vitamin B12 deficiency, and MALT lymphoma). In children, a similar attitude was obtained in all of these pathologies except for cITP, in which the investigation for *H. pylori* is not indicated.

**Keywords:** *Helicobacter pylori*, iron deficiency anemia, immune thrombocytopenia, MALT lymphoma, vitamin B12 deficiency

## 1. Introduction

*Helicobacter pylori* is a gram-negative spiral bacterium, responsible for one of the most frequent gastrodigestive infections in the world. In 1883, Bizzozero reported spirochetes inhabiting the gastric glands of dogs [1]. However, in 1954, after examining 1000 gastric biopsies, Palmer concluded that no microorganisms could survive in an acidic gastric environment [2]. This was contradicted by Marshall and Warren in 1982 [2].They isolated the microorganism from the specimens of gastric mucosa in patients with gastritis and peptic ulcers, and for the first time it was isolated in vitro culture. As previously stated, at that time, it was thought that the acidic gastric environment was not compatible with the survival of this bacterium. In 1991, an association between *H. pylori* infection and gastric mucosa-associated lymphoid tissue (MALT) lymphoma was found [3]. Then, in 1994, The National Institute of Health consensus conference in the United States declared an association between *H. pylori* infection and peptic ulcer disease [4]. In that same year, *H. pylori* was identified with gastric adenocarcinoma and gastric non-Hodgkin lymphoma [3, 4].

After the discovery made by Marshall and Warren, histological features of chronic gastritis in upper gastrointestinal endoscopy were revealed. Moreover, a Canadian group also found *H. pylori* in the gastric mucosa of children with gastritis and duodenal ulcers [5].

Although over 80% of infected subjects remain asymptomatic, *H. pylori* chronic infection is associated with different clinical manifestations, including chronic gastritis, peptic ulcer disease, lymphoid tissue (MALT) lymphoma, and gastric adenocarcinoma. Furthermore, in 1994, *H. pylori* was classified as a type 1 carcinogen by the World Health Organization (WHO) [6-8]. In children, *H. pylori* has been considered a cause of chronic gastritis and duodenal ulcers. Recently, it has been related to diseases outside the stomach, namely those characterized by persistent and low-grade systemic inflammation: iron deficiency anemia (IDA), chronic idiopathic thrombocytopenia (cITP), vitamin B12 deficiency, growth retardation, and diabetes mellitus [9, 10]. Although a relationship between the *H. pylori* infection and autoimmune atrophic gastritis (AAG) is not possible, studies conducted by Hershko proved that *H. pylori* can be the trigger of AAG and be responsible in the initial phase of the disease for an oral refractory iron anemia [11-14]. More debated hematological associations have been made with monoclonal gammopathy, non-Hodgkin lymphomas of the stomach, myelodysplastic syndromes, increased risk of childhood leukemia in the children of *H. pylori*-infected mothers, and gastric bleeding in children with coagulation pathologies [15-17].

The *H. pylori* infection is acquired during childhood (before the age of 10) and in the absence of antibiotic therapy the host can carry it for life. In contrast to the great majority of bacterial infections, in which virulence is temporary due to an immune system mechanism, which results in the clearance of the pathogen, *H. pylori* can survive for many years [15-18]. *H. pylori* has mechanisms to escape the clearance of the innate and adaptive immune system, and the development of a symbiotic relationship between the bacteria and the human host is also a possibility [9-12]. Moreover, *H. pylori* has an important urease activity, leading to ammonia production in order to protect itself from gastric acidity. Also, *H. pylori* produces enzymes, such as phospholipase A2 and C as well as glycosulphatase, which leads to gastric mucosa damage [6].

## 2. The interaction between *H. pylori* and the immune system

Epithelial and myeloid cells form the initial line of the innate immune system response against *H. pylori* infection. They recognize the bacteria through a limited number of microbial pattern recognition receptors (PRRs), which include membrane associated Toll like receptors (TLRs), cytoplasmic Nod-like receptors (NLRs) and retinoic acid inducible gene I-like helicase receptor (RLRs). They recognize bacteria constituents termed pathogen-associated molecular patterns (PAMPs), present in the microbial proteins, nucleic acids, lipids and carbohydrates. These PAMPs contain molecules that act as ligands to trigger PRRs dependent intracellular signaling pathways, inducting the expression of pro-inflammatory molecules and cytokines as the first response to the bacteria infection. TLRs are the most studied of the larger family of the PRRs and participate in the first line of host defense against pathogens, with subsequent activation of adaptive immune response [17-21]. Ten TLRs have been identified in humans and can be identified by the type of ligand [12-14]. TLRs are type I transmembrane proteins characterized by an extracellular leucine-rich ectodomain involved in PAMP recognition from bacteria, fungi, parasites, and viruses, including lipid components of wall cell bacteria such as lipopolysaccharides (LPS) and lipopeptides, microbial components such as flagellin and nucleic acid components, as well as an intracytoplasmatic domain that shows similarity to the IL1 receptor family termed a toll-IL1 receptor (TIR), which is involved in the activation of downstream signaling pathways. TLRs are expressed on the surface of cells or in intracellular vesicles like endosomes [18, 19, 22, 23]. Some TLRs recognize only one type of PAMP, while others such as TLR2 recognize bacterial lipoproteins, lipoteichoic acid and peptidoglycans [21]. The Goldberg Group revealed the role of TLRs during *H. pylori* infection, showing an overexpression of TLR2 and TLR5 in the gastric epithelial cells HEK293 of *H. pylori*-infected patients, as well as an increase of the activation of transcriptional factors: (1) nuclear factor-κB (NF-κB) and interleukin-8 (IL-8), (2) macrophage inflammatory protein 3$\alpha$ (MI-3$\alpha$), and (3) the growth-regulated protein-$\alpha$ (GRO-$\alpha$ mRNA expression) [8]. The understanding of the role of TLRs in response to *H. pylori* infection requires an elucidation of cell-signaling events. After PAMP recognition, TLRs trigger the signaling pathways resulting in: (1) activation of the transcription of NF-B, protein-1 (AP-1), and of interferon regulatory factors (IRFs); (2) increased expression of inflammatory cytokines, antimicrobial peptides, and interferon type 1 (INF-1); and (3) recruitment of neutrophils, activation of macrophage, and dendritic cells. In epithelial cells, studies have found an increased induction of pro-inflammatory genes caused by the interaction between *H. pylori* and 4TLR [18, 19, 22, 23].

MyD88 (myeloid differentiation primary response protein 88) is an intracellular adaptor protein used by all TLRs except TLR3, and the signaling is done in two forms: MyD88 dependent, responsible for pro-inflammatory cytokine production as well as MyD88 independent, responsible for interferon type 1 production (ITF1). TLR4 inducts both dependent and independent MyD88, so it inducts both cytokines and ITF1. The expression of MyD88 in macrophage cells is essential for the induction of anti-inflammatory cytokines (IL-6, IL-1B, IL-10, and IL-12) [19]. Recently, a new group of innate immune molecules, including activating receptors involved in modulating the intensity of innate immune response in myeloid cells (TREM), has been described [24, 25]. TREM family receptors (TREM-1 to TREM 4), are cell surface activating receptors with a transmembrane region containing charged lysine residues and a short cytoplasmatic tail lacking signaling motifs. TREM-1, a 30-Kda glycoprotein of the Ig family is the most well-known member of the TREM family and is responsible for inflammation amplification and activation of antigen-presenting cells (APC). TREM-1 is exhibited in neutrophils and monocytes and linked to innate immunity by phagocyte secretion of pro-inflammatory chemokines and cytokines such as IL-8 and TNF-$\alpha$. TREM-1 is involved in the amplification of TLR-dependent signals and in the improvement of NOD-like receptors (NLRs)–mediated responses, including NOD-1, involved in the protection against *H. pylori* infection [19]. An up-regulation of TREM-1 in gastric epithelial cells of *H. pylori* infected adults patients was found in a study by Schmausser et al. using immunohistochemistry in nine of twelve patients. No TREM-1 was found in non-inflamed gastric epithelium, in accordance with mRNA, TREM-1 also strongly expressed in *H. pylori* gastritis. [19, 26]. These results are not in accordance with Michalkiewics study done in 78 children with *H. pylori* infection. The gastric expression of TREM-1 and TREM-2 was not affected by H.pylori infection, reflecting the tolerance status of leucocytes present in gastric mucosa of H pylori infected children [19]. TREM-2 is expressed in macrophage and dendritic cells, acts antagonistically to TREM-1 and its activation results in anti-inflammatory reactions. This receptor has not yet been observed in *H. pylori*-infected patients. M1 macrophage cells are linked to strong pro-inflammatory and cytotoxic responses induced by INF$\gamma$, tumor necrosis factor (TNF), and IL-6. M2 macrophage cells show markers of an anti-inflammatory process through CD163, a cell surface glycoprotein whose expression is induced by inflammatory mediators, such as glucocorticoides and IL-10. Also, they are inhibited by pro-inflammatory mediators, such as INF$\gamma$, TNF-$\alpha$, as well as others [18, 19, 22, 23]. The CD14 receptor is a cell surface molecule expressed on monocytes and macrophages and linked to the recognition of *H. pylori* LPS, which leads to the production of many pro-inflammatory cytokines. The interaction of *H. pylori* and CD14 shows that its expression in gastric mucosa may indicate infiltration by monocytes/macrophages [27]. On the other hand, *H. pylori* has two major factors for virulence, vacuolating cytotoxin (VacA) and *H. pylori* neutrophil-activating protein (*H. pylori*-NAP), related to the stimulation of radical oxygen production by neutrophils. *H. pylori*-NAP is a 150-KDa oligomeric protein, a TLR2 agonist that exhibits chemotaxis for the neutrophils and monocytes, increasing the synthesis of tissue factor and type-2 plasminogen inhibitor, IL-23, and IL-12, a key cytokine for the differentiation of naïve T helper (TH) cells into the TH1 cytotoxic phenotype. Naïve T CD4+ helper TCD4+ cells can be called to differentiate towards TH1, TH2, TH17, and regulatory T cells (Tregs) phenotypes according to the cytokines. Classically, TH cells are divided into two functional subsets: Th1 and Th2, responsible for the production of a distinct pattern of cytokine secretion. The adaptive system produced by the host against *H. pylori* includes Th1 and Th17 components that are implicated in the control of infection. Despite these data, a number of reports suggest that this Th1-biased response is dysfunctional and can be considered as an important role in pathogenesis of *H. pylori*-related diseases [23, 27, 28]. Indeed the immuno-modulatory properties of the pathogen can reprogram the host's immune tolerance and *H. pylori* escapes [19]. In a study published by Michalkiewics, 78 children, ranging in ages between 7 and 18 years, with a confirmed *H. pylori* infection in 40 patients (50% without symptoms), a Th1 profile of *H. pylori*-mediated inflammation was found [28]. *H. pylori* can modulate MyD88 expression. In other words, the lack of significant amounts of MyD88 can explain the persistence of the infection and the endotoxin tolerance [19]. Furthermore, the exact role of T Helper cells in *H. pylori* infection is not fully understood. Recent studies revealed that a deficiency in Th1 response may be responsible for the persistence of *H. pylori* infection [28, 29]. The role of *H. pylori* in pathogenesis of extra-gastroduodenal diseases may be based on the systemic effects of chronic gastric inflammation immune responses, which can induce lesions outside of the stomach and can be reversed after *H. pylori* eradication [10, 14-16].

## 3. Epidemiology and risk factors

More than 50% of the world's population is infected with *H. pylori* [7, 8, 30]. Although infection occurs worldwide, its prevalence shows a marked discordance within and between developed and developing countries. Overall prevalence oscillates between 30 and 50% in industrialized countries, in contrast with the ranges of 80–90% found in the developing countries. Within geographic areas, the predominance correlates inversely with socioeconomic status, especially those related with living conditions during childhood. The improvement in hygiene, sanitary conditions, and the active treatment of the *H. pylori* carrierships implemented in developed countries may be the responsible for the difference in these two worlds [6, 7, 17, 31-34]. Reports regarding racial and ethnic differences in the prevalence of *H. pylori* infection in children and adults have been carried out. Everhart et al. reported an overall seropositivity rate of *H. pylori* infection in 32.7% of 7465 adult participants in the United States. Higher prevalence was observed in non-Hispanic blacks and Mexican Americans (51.1 and 57.9%, respectively), compared with the values observed among non-Hispanic whites (26.9%) [29]. A study conducted by Nguyen et al. in two ethnic groups (Kinh and Khmer), with different cultures, involving 1596 individuals, 485 households, the seroprevalence was higher in adults than in children ≤18 years (40.2 and 32.1%, respectively). Variables related to promiscuity such as taking foods by hands, absence of good practice of hand washing after defecation, having mother or siblings infected by *H. pylori* were risk factors. There were no differences in *H. pylori* seropositivity based on sex ($P>0.05$) or ethnicity ($P>0.05$) [31]. In southern China, the prevalence of *H. pylori* infection in Chinese people was significantly higher than in Australians (44.2 vs. 21%). Comparing the prevalence of infection in children aged <10 years, the Chinese showed 27% and the Australians 4%. In children over the age of 10, a similar rate of *H. pylori* acquisition was observed in both countries (1% per annum), according to epidemiological data [32]. Cherian conducted a cross-sectional study in 193 African refugee children (aged <16 years) in Western Australia. The mean age was 7.9 years, and 18 children (9%, mean age of 11.3 months, and SD 5.2 months) were breastfeeding. There were 116 children living in refugee camps and the remaining lived in apartments or houses. The great majority came from Tanzania or Kenya, 96 of 97 (99%), lived in the camps, whereas 28 originating from Egypt lived in apartments and houses. *H. pylori* was present in 82% of children (63% aged <2 years), rising to 95% for those older than 14 years, confirming a greater risk in Africa. Intrafamilial spread of *H. pylori*, particularly mother-to-child transmission or infected older siblings, was a potential mechanism of this acquisition. Concerning the breastfeeding children, a statistically significant correlation was not possible because the number of children was small. Curiously, those children who had done antimalarial treatment seemed to have eradicated *H. pylori*. It was attributed to a probable effect of artemisinin on the iron dependence of the bacteria [33]. Differences in the prevalence of *H. pylori* infection among racial and ethnic groups have been described. Besides ethnicity, the difference in the prevalence between developed and developing countries seems to be linked to socioeconomic factors. Poverty and bad living conditions are the principle risk factors for acquiring *H. pylori* infection within industrialized countries [6-8, 34-36]. A high number of residents in the same home, sharing the same room or the same bed with *H. pylori*-infected children, as well as poor sanitary conditions were identified as major risk factors [6-8]. This infection is acquired in childhood and they are carrying the same strain as their parents and maintain this genotype even after moving to a different environment [37, 38]. In relation to the prevalence based on gender, differences have not been found between men and women, and no association with smoking or drinking habits has been made [6]. Nutritional status has been described as being associated to *H. pylori* infection. Goodman et al. found reduced odds of risk of *H. pylori* infection in adults and children with an increased ingestion of fruit, vegetables, and milk. The increased improvement of hygiene at home, as well as socioeconomic conditions, has resulted in a lower rate of *H. pylori* infection and an increase of gastroesophageal reflux disease (GERD) [8, 32, 35-37]. Studies revealed that gastric corpus inflammation induced by *H. pylori*, more pronounced with CagA+ strains, has an acid-suppressive effect, preventing the development of GERD. Also, asthma and allergy disorders are prevalent in developed countries and inversely associated with *H. pylori* [8, 14-16, 33, 34, 36]. Hygiene reduces the exposures to microorganism modifiers polarized Th1/Th2 responses leading to asthma. *H. pylori* can alter the polarized Th1/Th2 through dendritic cell-mediated T expression of IL-2, TNF-$\alpha$, and INF-$\gamma$. Longitudinal studies revealed that asthma is a risk factor to GERD development and GERD can trigger asthma [36, 37]. The most well-known hematological pathology linked to *H. pylori* infection in children is IDA. Epidemiological studies have indicated that seropositivity is associated to low serum ferritin and hemoglobin levels compared with seronegative controls. Reports have been carried out concerning refractory iron deficiency anemia (refractory IDA), normalized after the *H. pylori* eradication therapy and also the improvement of anemia without iron supplementation [11-13].

### 3.1. Routes of transmission

A number of studies propose environmental sources, such as animal and water exposure, as potential forms of *H. pylori* infection. Also, a human-to-human transmission through oral-oral, fecal-oral, or both has been described. *H. pylori* has been detected in saliva, vomitus, gastric reflux, and feces [6, 8, 33, 34, 39-42].

#### *3.1.1. Animals as potential source of H. pylori*

Two epidemiological studies reported that the exposure to sheep was implicated in *H. pylori* infection. Goodman et al. [35] described a higher risk of *H. pylori* infection, in the Colombian Andes, in children who played with sheep. Dore et al. reported an association between a prevalence of infection in 98% of Sardinian shepherds and the contact with sheep and sheepdogs. In that study, the individuals had a significant increase of infection prevalence not observed in their family members, with no regular contact with sheep (73%) or sheepdogs (43%). A subsequent recovery of *H. pylori* in sheep milk led Dore to suggest that *H. pylori* may be a commensal of sheep and thus the last ancestral host of *H. pylori*. The isolation of *H. pylori* in the stomach of cats led Handt et al. to suggest that cats may also represent a reservoir of the bacteria [27, 29, 43]. Rothenbacher et al. found that adults, who owned cats as children, had a higher prevalence of *H. pylori* infection. Contradicting these studies were El-Zaatari et al. who reported, in 25 stray cats, no infection by *H. pylori*. They found another strain, *Helicobacter heilmannii* to be responsible for chronic gastritis in cats. Two seroepidemiological studies in the United States, involving pet owners, failed to support the association of the relationship between pet owners and an increased prevalence of *H. pylori* [32]. One large population-based study in Canada, adjusted for social class, found no association between pet ownership and peptic ulcer disease. With these results, a relation between cats and *H. pylori* infection does not seem possible, and cats are not a health problem for cat owners [34].

#### 3.1.2. Water transmission

*H. pylori* can survive for several days in milk and tap water in an infectious bacillary form. In rivers, it can survive in a coccoid form for several months. Under physical or chemical stress, *H. pylori* is capable of converting into a viable form. It is not known whether this coccoid form can revert to its infectious form. Several studies support this form of transmission [34, 39, 40, 44]. In 1993, Westbloom detected *H. pylori* in the sewage water in Peru [6]. Hulten et al. showed that in a population of Peruvian children, which consumed an internal source of water at home, the likelihood of having infection with *H. pylori* was tripled [39]. In Colombia, children who swam in rivers, streams, and pools and drank from a stream contaminated with sewage water had a higher tendency of acquiring the infection. In South America, Hopkins et al. found, in Chilean children who consumed uncooked vegetables contaminated with water containing raw sewage, an increased prevalence of the infection [33-35].

#### 3.1.3. Fecal-oral transmission

Some studies support the evidence of the transmission of *H. pylori* through its elimination in feces after turnover of gastric mucosa. Thomas et al. in 1992 detected it in the feces of one adult and 9 of 23 children living in a Gambian village, using the culture method. The isolation of *H. pylori* from feces has been controversial. Parsonnet et al. [41] cultured the bacteria in feces, in 7 of 14 *H. pylori*-infected adults after cathartic-induced diarrhea. Mapstone et al. in 1993 detected *H. pylori* DNA by polymerase chain reaction (PCR). Some studies reported detection of *H. pylori* by DNA, in feces, in 25–90% of *H. pylori*-infected patients [34]. In 1993, Hopkins et al. observed that the consumption of fertilized vegetables with human feces was a risk factor for acquiring *H. pylori* infection. The spreading through feces is supported by the occurrence of infection in institutionalized people during gastroenteritis outbreaks [8, 34].

#### 3.1.4. Oral-oral transmission

It is accepted that *H. pylori* infection acquisition occurs in early childhood by close interfamilial contact. Many scientists report that oral-oral transmission is the most common form in developed countries. This was supported by the high prevalence of *H. pylori* infection observed in institutionalized people, within families, and in dentists. Megraud found, in Western Africa, a higher risk of *H. pylori* infection in children fed with premasticated foods by their parents [34]. Parsonnet et al. [41] isolated *H. pylori* from saliva, vomitus, and cathartic stools in 16 healthy volunteers, infected adults, using culture and PCR methods. Ferguson et al. also demonstrated by PCR, a low number of *H. pylori* from the saliva in one of the nine *H. pylori*-positive subjects. By using soluble electrophoresis on polyacrylamide slab gels, restriction endonuclease analysis, and Southern blot hybridization, they confirmed that the same strain was isolated from both saliva and gastric biopsy [42]. In 1993, Mapstone detected *H. Pylori* in the oral cavity, by culture, in one person. Majmudar et al. using PCR diagnosed *H. pylori* in dental plaque [6, 8]. Cellini et al. reported the isolation of *H. pylori* from the dental plaque of 1 in 20 *H. pylori*-positive patients. Comparing the protein patterns and the restriction endonuclease pattern of the bacteria, those isolated from gastric biopsy and from dental plaque showed to be identical [32]. Peach et al. found an association between *H. pylori* infection with a high plaque score. However, studies conducted by other investigators did not find a relationship between dentist visits, number of times that teeth were brushed, and periodontal status. Doré-Davin et al. found no correlation between *H. pylori* infection, determined by PCR, on saliva and dental plaque. They state that the transmission was done by gastro-esophageal reflux or regurgitation of gastric contents [34, 41, 42].

## 4. Pathogenesis of *H. pylori* infection in extradigestive pathologies

It is known that the immunological response triggered by the bacteria is responsible for gastric mucosa damage. Large amounts of pro-inflammatory substances, such as cytokines, eicosanoids, and acute phase proteins, are released after *H. pylori* colonization [14-19]. Also, cross mimicry between bacteria and host antigens may contribute to gastric mucosa damage [8, 22]. Although *H. pylori* gastric colonization induces histological changes in gastric mucosa, leading to chronic gastritis in all infected people, most have no symptoms. The risk of developing symptoms will depend on factors, such as the interaction between the host and the bacterium, host genetic and immune response, diet and level of gastric acid. Host immune gene polymorphisms and gastric acid secretion determine the bacterium's ability to colonize a specific gastric niche. Some bacteria strains are more virulent than others. The increase of pathogenicity is related to the induction of morphological changes, vacuolation, and successive degeneration of cells in vitro. The protein vacuolating cytotoxin VacA and the cytotoxin-associated gene pathogenicity island-encoded protein CagA seem to be essential for the colonization and for modulating the host's immune system. The pathogen effects of *H. pylori* are related to chronic inflammation, with the promotion of pro-inflammatory and anti-inflammatory mediators. Host genetics polymorphisms can affect the expression levels of these mediators [8].

### 4.1. Pathogenesis of *H. pylori* in extradigestive disorders

The role of *H. pylori* in the pathogenesis of extradigestive disorders is based on (1) local inflammation has systemic effects, (2) *H. pylori* infection is a chronic process that persists for several decades, and (3) the persistent infection induces a chronic inflammatory and immune response that can induce lesions locally and remote to the primary site of infection [14]. In addition to the above, several reports have revealed the role of *H. pylori* infection in hematological problems [10, 16, 45]. Unexplained ID, IDA, and cITP are the most common problems encountered in pediatric groups [11, 16]. Vitamin B12 (vit.B12) deficiency was the first hematological disease associated to *H. pylori* infection and considered an elderly age group's disease. A study conducted by Rogers et al. for the evaluation of risk factors contributing to low or marginal vitamin B12 concentration in Guatemalan school children revealed that malabsorption conditions can interfere with vitamin uptake of the diet. A normal vitamin B12 status is expected despite a low intake because of this efficient enterohepatic circulation. An additional hypo/achlorhydria produced by *H. pylori* infection can be the trigger to the development of cyanocobalamin deficiency in this young age group [46].

Gastric MALT lymphoma, also known as mucosa-associated lymphoid tissue (lymphoma), is a low grade B-cell lymphoma described by Isaac and Wright in 1993 as an adult disease and extremely rare in children. *H. pylori* stimulates the B and T lymphocytes of the stomach. B cells form clones, possibility by trissomia-3 mutations, and can become low-grade MALT lymphoma. The *H. pylori* dependence is by-passed to *H. pylori* independence with genetic mutations t(1:14) with a transformation to high-grade MALT lymphoma, not documented in children [9, 47, 48].

The Scientific community has discussed and incorporated international consensus guidelines for investigation and management of these hematological extragastric pathologies (IDA, cITP, vitamin B12 deficiency, and MALT lymphoma) [5, 49-51]. No international consensus was obtained for other hematological changes. However, autoimmune neutropenia was documented in 2002 by Gupta et al. [52] with the report of a patient with a neutropenia (400/µl), which normalized after *H. pylori* eradication. Papadaki et al. [53] in 2006, after evaluating 67 adult patients with chronic neutropenia and splenomegaly, found a higher prevalence of *H. pylori* infection compared to healthy controls.

According to literature, other hematologic problems may be associated to *H. pylori* infection. For example, leukemia in children, whose mothers are chronic carriers of *H. pylori*, increased risk of gastric bleeding in children with acute leukemia, *H. pylori* infected, and in patients with genetic diseases prone to hemorrhage (Hemophilia A and B and thrombasthenia) [15, 16].

## 5. Iron deficiency anemia

The World Health Organization (WHO) estimates that approximately 50% of all anemic patients have a diagnosis of IDA [1, 30, 31, 50, 51, 54]. In infancy, IDA is associated to abnormal mental and motor development. In developed countries, low intake, increased host requirements to supply the physiological needs for normal development, dietary errors, and blood loss are the most frequent causes of IDA in children [15, 45]. The evidence to support a causal association between *H. pylori* infection and ID or IDA is based on epidemiological studies and clinical trials. The first clinical case was described by Becker in 1991, in a 15-year-old girl, *H. pylori* positive, whose clinical presentation was a chronic active hemorrhagic gastritis, without gastrointestinal symptoms. In 1993, Dufour et al. reported a 7-year-old child without evidence of hemorrhage or clinical symptoms, with refractory IDA to oral iron therapy. The investigation revealed an *H. pylori*-positive patient. High endoscopy showed chronic antral gastritis and *H. pylori* eradication reversed the anemia [55]. These case reports were followed by other studies that have documented an association between *H. pylori* infection and unexplained or refractory IDA with reversal of anemia and a normalization of iron stores after successful *H. pylori* eradication, with or without iron supplementation [10, 45]. A recurrent ID or an inadequate response to oral iron therapy implies searching for *H. pylori* infection. All guidelines and international consensus support that *H. pylori* should be sought and eradicated in ID cases [5, 49, 50, 56].

### 5.1. Pathophysiology of iron deficiency by *H. pylori*

The intrinsic biological mechanisms by which *H. pylori* infection induces ID, IDA, or refractory IDA are not fully understood. However, several pathways are involved: occult blood loss, changes in gastric physiology as the result of chronic gastric inflammation and of low gastric acidity and ascorbate, as well as mechanisms used by the bacteria for its growth [11-13, 55].

#### *5.1.1. Occult blood loss*

Chronic gastrointestinal blood loss is one of the supposed intrinsic mechanisms. However, most case series of *H. pylori* patients with anemia and chronic gastritis do not reveal gastric bleeding lesions at the time of endoscopy, and positive occult fecal blood tests are not always present [45, 57]. The occult fecal blood test is a qualitative and highly accurate (98%) form of detecting human fecal hemoglobin, based on a flow chromatographic immunoassay, it is a diagnostic approach for the evaluation of gastrodigestive pathology of detecting human fecal hemoglobin, based on a flow chromatographic immunoassay [58]. A literature review by Susan Owens et al. about gastrointestinal bleeding in children, considered the *H. pylori* infection in children with hemorrhagic hereditary disorders, such as hemophilia A and B as a risk factor for severe hemorrhage [16]. Also, Campuzano-Maya mentioned that an increased risk of hemorrhage is observed in patients with acute leukemia infected with *H. pylori*, which have a greater risk of gastrointestinal hemorrhage during treatment compared to uninfected patients. This risk is reduced if a screening and eradication therapy, is offered to all leucemia patients upon starting leucemia treatment if they are infected [16] Therefore, in patients with potentially hemorrhagic genetic diseases, such as hemophilias (A and B) and Von Willebrand disease, *H. pylori* infection should be considered as an important cause of upper gastrointestinal bleeding. The authors recommend a stool antigen test as a new and non-invasive screening test for diagnosing *H. pylori* infection in all patients with hereditary hemorrhagic disorders [16].

#### *5.1.2. Changes in gastric physiology: gastric inflammation and chronic disease anemia*

Gastric mucosal inflammation is an invariable finding in *H. pylori*-infected patients and represents the host's immune response to the bacteria [59]. Several mechanisms have been postulated: (a) directed mucosal injury enhancing permeability and the antigen exposure; (b) adherence of bacteria to the gastric mucosal, accompanied by microvilli loss, irregularity of luminal border, edema and vacuolation; (c) toxic effect of the bacteria on epithelial cells with a gastric epithelial degeneration, access to underlying mucosa, stimulating host non-specific and specific responses involving several cytokines' liberation [59].

#### *5.1.2.1. Directed mucosal injury*

Two instances should be considered in the invasion of *H. pylori* in gastric mucosal. In the first, *H. pylori* colonizes, living in the mucus layer in proximity to the epithelial surface. This interaction leads to epithelial cell damage and liberation of pro-inflammatory cytokines [8, [59].

#### *5.1.2.2. Adherence of bacteria to the gastric mucosal*

After the initial colonization, *H. pylori* migrates to the mucosa with stimulation of immune responses. All *H. pylori* strains have the gene for vacuolation cytotoxin (VacA), but only 50% produce the VacA protein, capable of vacuolation eukaryotic cells and prone to insertion into the membranes of endosomal vesicles forming pores with chloride channel activity. This alters the anions' composition within the endosomes, which leads to osmotic swelling, cellular death and apoptosis, and a more severe degree of inflammation and peptic ulceration [59].

#### *5.1.2.3. Toxic effect*

Several enzymes produced by *H. pylori* may contribute to changes in gastric mucosa permeability. *H. pylori* is one of the most powerful urea-splitting organisms. Splitting urea leads to the release of nitrogen and ammonia, increasing the pH of the gastric antrum, one of the mechanisms that protects the bacteria from the gastric acidity and has a toxic effect on the mucosa. Bacterial phospholipases can destroy gastric mucosa phospholipids, and acetaldehyde dehydrogenase production may have also a toxic mucosal effect [59].

### *5.1.3. Recruitment of inflammatory chemokines and inflammatory cells*

*H. pylori* is a non-invasive bacterium. However, after the initial phase of the colonization, a dense infiltration of granulocytes begins and it is followed, in the chronic phase, by a predominant infiltration of plasma cells and lymphocytes. It seems that signal transduction pathways must exist in order to induce the recruitment and immigration of inflammatory cells to the gastric mucosa. Additionally, soluble bacterial products may initiate the inflammatory cascade [17, 60]. Gastric *H. pylori* infection is associated to the epithelium release of several chemokines [60, 61]. Each chemokine is involved in the recruitment and activation of a specific immune cell. Potential chemoattractants of the CXC chemokine family, IL-8, GRO-$\alpha$, and epithelial cell–derived neutrophil-activating protein 78 (ENA-78), are involved in the recruitment of neutrophils. Members of the C-C family (RANTES, MIP- 1$\alpha$) have specificity for monocyte and lymphocyte recruitment. IL 8 expression has been detected in epithelial cells of antral biopsy and in the supernatant of antral biopsy samples in *H. pylori*-infected patients [59, 60]. *H. pylori* induces gastric epithelial cells to increase transcription and secretion of IL 8. TNF-$\alpha$ has an effect on leukocyte activation, and IL7 has a regulating role on lymphocytes B and T [59]. Studies state that cytokine levels, with a pro-inflammatory effect, such as IL-6, IL-8, and TNF-$\alpha$ are higher in *H. pylori*-positive patients than in *H. pylori* negative [49]. Among these,

IL-6 is the most important pro-inflammatory cytokine inductor of the hepcidin gene transcription through STAT3 (signal transducer and activator of transcription 3) [61, 62]. Hepcidin is a small peptide hormone primarily expressed in hepatocytes as a propeptide precursor. Prohepcidin is processed to a bioactive molecule of 25 amino acids, the hepcidin that is secreted into the blood stream and eliminated in urine. Hepcidin is the most important regulator of iron homeostasis [63, 64]. The expression of hepcidin is regulated on a transcriptional level by two principal pathways. The first is the activation of STAT 3. Upon activation, these proteins are transferred to the nucleus where they activate transcription of the hepcidin gene, binding to a sequence of DNA. The second is transcription control dependent on the BMP/Smad pathway, which involves Smad proteins and bone morphogenetic proteins (BMPs). Factors that can affect the expression of hepcidin are iron, anemia, hypoxia, and inflammation [61-68]. Hepcidin is a negative regulator of a transmembrane protein, ferroportin, which is expressed on the surface of all cells that release iron in circulation: enterocytes, macrophages, hepatocytes, and placental cells. Hepcidin regulates ferroportin at a translational level [67]. Under inflammatory conditions, hepcidin reacts as an acute reagent phase, increasing its expression, binding to ferroportin for tyrosine phosphorylation and also the internalization and ubiquitin-mediated degradation in lysosomes, resulting in hypoferremia and no iron availability for erythropoiesis, the hallmark of inflammatory anemia. In 1932, Locke et al. observed that infection was associated with low serum iron levels [63, 64]. This finding was corroborated by Cartwright and Wintrobe with the demonstration that anemia associated with infection was not different from anemia of inflammation, resulting in a pathology known as anemia of inflammation or chronic disease anemia [63, 68]. On the other hand, *H. pylori* can subvert human iron to benefit itself instead of the host, and recently hepcidin has been identified in the parietal cells of *H. pylori*-infected patients with an upregulated gastric hepcidin and a consequent downregulation of ferroportin [63, 67, 69].

### *5.1.4. Hypochlorhydria*

Iron absorption takes place in the small intestine in accordance with the metabolic demands that reflect the amount of iron stored for erythropoiesis. Haem iron refers to the pool of iron incorporated in the protoporfirin ring. Its absorption is more effective than non-haem iron and the mechanisms for absorption are different. HCP 1 (haem carrier protein) is a protein capable of the transmembrane transport of haem into the lumen of enterocytes to be catabolized by the microsomal enzyme haem oxygenase. The non-haem iron ($Fe^{3+}$) is not soluble and is the most prevalent alimentary iron. Its absorption is dependent on endogenous factors related to its reduction to a soluble iron form ($Fe2^{+}$), such as duodenal cytochrome *b* reductase, and the ascorbic acid released by gastric cells [70]. Gastric acidity increases the absorption of $Fe^{3+}$ in two ways: (1) the high concentration of hydrogen ions at acidic pH (pH 3 = 1 mM $H^{+}$) leads to an efficient competition for metal iron in bindings sites, on dietary components; (2) mechanisms related with the release of soluble ferric ions only in acidic pH ($pH<4$) [71]. In 1905, John Edkins postulated gastrin as the hormone regulator for gastric acid secretion [72]. Sarker et al. [65] revealed that the basal and stimulated gastric acid was greatly reduced in *H. pylori*-infected children compared to non-infected [10, 16, 71]]. The same author revealed, in a study with *H. pylori*-infected children of Bangladesh, that this infection was associated to impaired gastric secretion. After *H. pylori* eradication, improved gastric secretion and hemoglobin concentration was observed but no influence on iron absorption was verified. Other possible mechanism such as competition for oral iron and inflammatory disease was considered a possibility. A study performed by Harris in 105 children, 33 *H. pylori* positive and 72 *H. pylori* negative, found a significantly higher percentage of *H. pylori*-infected children with a gastric juice pH above 4.0 (6/33, 18%) compared to *H. pylori*-negative children (6/10, 60%) [70]. While hypochlorhydria and acute *H. pylori* infection in adults is well documented, the mechanisms inducting hypochlorhydria in children are not well understood [8, 10, 16, 70]. *H. pylori* can induce hypochlorhydria through increased gastric IL-1β and TNF-α, both in adults and in children, which inhibits acid gastric secretion, induces parietal apoptosis, and decreases enterochromafin-like cell histamine release [10, 70]. Capurso et al. [67] demonstrated that *H. pylori*-infected IDA patients, with involvement of corporal gastric mucosa, had an important decrease of gastric acidity (pH>4) with higher intragastric pH and high serum gastrin levels. Serum gastrin is an indirect marker of atrophic gastritis [11, 12, 73]. As described by Hartmann et al., iron malabsorption can be confirmed by an oral iron challenge. In fast, 2 mg of iron sulfate is administrated, and the dosing of iron serum is done before ingestion and then after the first, second, and third hour. It is considered poor absorption when at the first hour the iron serum level is <100 μg/ml (Figure 1) [74]. Recently, *H. pylori* has been implicated in unexplained refractory IDA to oral iron treatment. This refractoriness may be defined as a failure of the hemoglobin increase at least 1 g/dL after 2 months of treatment [13]. Celiac disease is the most known pathology related with malabsorption conditions. AAG, manifested as hypergastrinemia, with strongly positive antiparietal cell antibodies, was for many years considered a disease of older people and vitamin B12 deficiency the only possible presentation. The age, gender, and severity of the disease are determinants for the presentation in microcytic or macrocytic anemia [11-13]. Although atrophic gastritis may impair both vitamin B12 and iron, the increase in the iron demands for the observed growth in children and adolescents as well as the menstrual blood loss in pubescent females, make IDA easier to develop. *H. pylori* can trigger AAG by a molecular mimicry between the bacteria and H+ K+-ATPase. In children, a refractory IDA without evidence of gastrointestinal blood loss implies in first line, non-invasive tests for Celiac disease (anti-endomysial antibodies IgG and IgA), AAG (serum gastrin in fasting and anti-parietal cells antibodies), and *H. pylori* infection (*H. pylori* IgG antibodies followed by urease breath test) [11-13]. IDA in the AAG context was described by Faber in 1909 and then completely ignored and forgotten. The role of *H. pylori* in AAG development is not consensual because of the high prevalence of this bacteria in the world population. However, eradication of *H. pylori* in this context is accompanied by a normalization of hemoglobin, iron stores, and gastrin levels [13, 16, 75].

#### *5.1.5. Low ascorbic acid level*

Vitamin C is an acidic molecule with strong reducing activity. Ascorbic acid (AA) is the reduced form of vitamin C. It is a potent antioxidant, a protector against gastric carcinogenesis, neutralizing nitrite-derived mutagens. Vitamin C is essentially absorbed and secreted in the antral mucosa. It has two major redox forms: AA and dehydroascorbic acid (DHA), the reduced

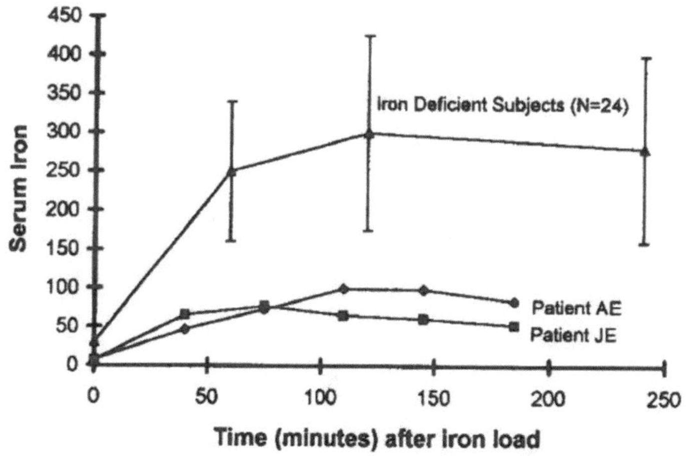


**Figure 1.** Oral iron challenge study. At the time, 0.2 mg/kg of elemental iron as ferrous sulfate was given. The expected normal response range, derived from 24 iron-deficient children but with normal absorption after given an oral dose of 1 mg /kg of elemental iron. Adapted with permission from Hartman and Barker [74]. Copyright ©1996.

and oxidized forms, respectively, and interconvertible. Within the cell, DHA is rapidly converted to AA by the specific enzyme systems, such as DHA reductase, glutaredoxins, and protein disulfide isomerase, in the presence of glutathione or other thiols as electron donors [76, 77]. Unlike AA, DHA is relatively unstable and undergoes rapid, spontaneous, and irreversible hydrolysis particularly at pH>4. Annibale et al. [73] demonstrated that gastric juice and ascorbate content are negatively affected by *H. pylori* infection and a normalization of ascorbate and gastric pH was obtained with eradication therapy [11-13, 78]. In *H. pylori*–infected children, a reduced gastric juice ascorbic acid concentration was found, and this effect was more evident in patients with CagA-positive strains [10, 30, 66, 71, 77]. A Korean study with the involvement of 452 patients (228 boys, 224 girls) aged 1–15 years revealed a negative correlation between gastric vitamin C level, *H. pylori* concentration, and the degree of active inflammation in antral mucosa. In this group, data showed that vitamin C levels in whole blood, plasma and gastric juice as well as the intragastric pH were closely related to the severity of the *H. pylori* infection and the histological changes in the stomach. These findings suggest that vitamin C may play a role in determining infection and progression [76, 79]. Studies have demonstrated that *H. pylori* produces gastric vitamin C reduction, promoting its degradation to DHA, a metabolite that may be oxidized at an irreversible form. This is unstable at high pH values, and thus hypochlorhydria reduces the bioavailability of this vitamin, essential for iron reduction to ferrous form, which forms an absorbable molecular complex with ferric iron, insoluble at pH>5 [10, 30, 45, 80]. Baysoy et al. documented a greater decrease in gastric juice ascorbate in *H. pylori*-infected patients with CagA-positive strains compared to those with CagA-negative strains [10, 45, 70, 71]. However, in this group, no association among CagA-positive strains and IDA has been found.

http://dx.doi.org/10.5772/63827

#### *5.1.6. Utilization/sequestering iron by H. pylori*

*H. pylori*, like other pathogenic bacteria, requires iron as a growth factor [8]. However, *H. pylori* does not produce siderophores capable of extracting iron from proteins. Potential iron sources for *H. pylori* are transferrin, lactoferrin, ferritin, hemosiderin, heme, and iron-containing enzymes [3, 81]. Lactoferrin is a source of iron for *H. pylori* in gastric mucosa. Choe et al. reported an abnormal elevated lactoferrin level in the stomachs of 101 adolescents with unexplained epigastric pain, ID, and *H. pylori* positive [10, 45, 82, 83]. A concordance was obtained with studies published by Dogan et al. [83] related to the gastric issues of 61 children with recurrent abdominal pain, 45 of which were *H. pylori* positive. It is known that lactoferrin captures iron from transferrin. *H. pylori* has a highly specific lactoferrin-binding protein. Thus, iron bound to lactoferrin is directed to *H. pylori*. The bacteria have a 19 KDa iron-binding protein that resembles ferritin, storing the iron, and making it unavailable for erythropoiesis [8, 67].

#### *5.1.7. Inhibitor effect on duodenal mucosa cells*

Duodenal mucosa cells are responsible for iron absorption. *H. pylori* can exert an inhibitor effect on the duodenal mucosa [8, 10].

### 5.2. Diagnosis

Symptoms of *H. pylori* infection in children are non-specific and can include: abdominal pain after meals, unexplained anorexia, nausea, recurrent vomiting, hematemesis, and IDA. These symptoms are considered to be of low predictive value. A meta-analysis of 45 studies concluded that *H. pylori* infection is not associated with abdominal pain. Therefore, an *H. pylori* infection diagnosing test for abdominal pain is not recommended as the first step of investigation [5, 49, 50, 56, 84]. In contrary, in a briefing for the European Gastroenterology Review, Mafertheiner et al. recommend that in children with a family history of peptic ulcer and gastric cancer, a recurrent abdominal pain should be subjected to testing for *H. pylori* after exclusion of other causes [49]. Based on the development of a chronic pangastritis with a consequent achlorhydria and reduced ascorbic acid, interference with iron absorption, occult blood loss by erosive gastritis or peptic ulcers, competition for the alimentary iron and sequestering by the bacteria, it seems reasonable to recommend testing for *H. pylori* infection on unexplained ID or IDA. Evidence-based guidelines from European Society for Pediatrics, Gastroenterology, Hepatology and Nutrition (ESPGHAN) and the Group of the North American Society for Pediatric Gastroenterology (NASPGHAN) in 2011 for IDA in context of *H. pylori* infection in children are in accordance with the Canadian Group Consensus Conference in 1999 [5, 49, 50]. They recommend considering diagnostic tests in children with refractory IDA, after the exclusion of other causes and in children with first-degree relatives with gastric cancer. In 2007, the American College of Gastroenterology, in their guidelines for the management of *H. pylori* infection, questioned this conclusion. Large studies from North America have reported that *H. pylori* infection was an independent risk factor for IDA in 688 school-aged children from Alaska and 7462 children, adolescents, and adults, all from the United States. A recent unblended study of 219 *H. pylori*-infected children, aged between 7 and 11 years, also from

Alaska, with pretreatment ID, found no difference in the likelihood of iron deficiency or anemia at 2 months or 14 months following a 6-week course of oral iron and antibiotics or no antibiotics. These data points support an association between *H. pylori* infection and IDA, but do not prove cause and effect. On the other hand, most studies refer to a relationship between *H. pylori* infection and IDA as well as a normalization with eradication therapy [11-13, 16, 49]. Antibody tests for *H. pylori* infection using whole blood, serum, and saliva are not recommended because of the low prevalence of *H. pylori*-related diseases in children and low specificity and sensitivity of the testes [51, 84].

## 6. Idiopathic thrombocytopenia purpura (ITP)

Immune thrombocytopenic purpura (ITP) is an autoimmune hemorrhagic disease, characterized by isolated thrombocytopenia, which affects nearly 1:25000 children per year [85-87]. ITP can present itself as an acute, self-limiting condition or a chronic process. Persistent thrombocytopenia, for longer than 6 months, may be present in about 20% of children [88-91]. A controversial issue in children is the designation "Chronic immune thrombocytopenia (cITP)," because about a third of children with ITP spontaneously cure from 6 months to 1 year later [87-89]. The International Childhood ITP Study Group recommends that 12 months must be the cutoff point for defining cITP [88, 90]. ITP is characterized by a premature destruction of platelets. Autoantibodies interact with the glycoprotein membrane on surface platelets (GIIb/IIIa or GIb), resulting in accelerated platelet destruction and clearance by mononuclear phagocytes [86, 91-93]. Increased megakaryocyte number in bone marrow is the marker of ITP in childhood [91]. However, studies performed in 1980 revealed that in two thirds of adults the expected increase of megakaryocyte production was not observed. Most of ITP had normal or depressed platelets turnover [87]. Chang et al. evaluated the effect of plasma, from childhood patients with ITP (44 with an acute form and 9 with chronic ITP), on induced thromboietin production of megakaryocytes in liquid culture. They reported that plasma from pediatric patients with ITP suppressed in vitro megakaryocyte production. They cultured cord blood cells as a source of CD34+ cells, which is a thrombopoietic growth factor, and plasma from control subjects or, children with ITP. After 8 days of culture, nearly 16% of cells were megakaryocytes. The effect of plasma in three groups was compared: control plasma, antibody ITP plasma (anti-GPIb, anti-GPIIIa, or both). They observed that in cultures with anti-GPIb antibodies the number of megakaryocytes were strongly reduced but this did not occur in ITP plasma negative antibody or in ITP plasma with only anti-GPIIb-IIIa antibody [93, 94]. Recently, thrombocyte kinetic studies have been carried out and autoantibodies affecting the megakaryocytes production in the bone marrow were observed [87, 91, 93, 95]. Also, studies using electronic microscopy showed 50–75% of ITP megakaryocytes damaged and in some cases attached by monocytes [96]. In most cases, ITP in childhood is triggered by a previous viral disease or a vaccination [87, 90]. HIV, hepatitis C, measles, cytomegalovirus, varicella, pertussis, and parvovirus can all be found in this context [95, 97]. After a benign viral infection, a predominant proinflammatory state may trigger ITP. Both proinflammatory cytokines and T-cells persist, creating a permissive environment for the emergence of autoantibodies that bind to platelet membrane antigens [91, 93]. Zehnder et al. highlighted an increased expression of gamma interferon-dependent genes in early states of ITP, supporting a proinflammatory or TH1 profile [91, 95]. ITP affects both adults and children. However, the natural course of ITP in children is different from adults. Spontaneous recovery occurs in one third of the pediatric patients, months or years after the diagnosis. Several studies in adults reported improvement in platelet counts after *H. pylori* eradication therapy [91, 98, 99]. Few studies exist related to children and the ones that do exist have contradictory findings. In a study developed in Taiwan, Jaing et al. evaluated 22 cITP children *H. pylori* infected, after one or two courses of eradication therapy. They found that 55.6% of patients experienced total or partial remission after an average of 16 months. In the Netherlands, a study carried out by Niefjes et al. evaluated 47 children with cITP, 3 of them *H. pylori* infected. They were treated with a 2-week course of triple therapy and after 6 months all of them acquired complete remission. In an Iranian study by Hamidieh et al., 31 cITP children were evaluated. Four of them were *H. pylori* infected and treated with 2 weeks of triple therapy. None of them acquired partial or complete remission. In Italy, Bisogno et al. evaluated 25 children with cITP. Nine of them were *H. pylori* infected and treated with 1–2 courses of 2 weeks of triple therapy. After 6 months, three patients had an increase in platelet counts and one had remission. This author also reported complete remission in 16 *H. pylori*-negative patients. The follow-up of the last 10 *H. pylori*-negative patients presented a platelet count above $50{\times}10^9$ without any treatment [10, 45]. Several studies revealed a widely variable prevalence among different populations according to the countries' epidemiology. In Finnish populations, *H. pylori* was not found in any of the 17 pediatric patients [100]. Turkish children showed *H. pylori* infection in 11 of 35 children (31%). Japan reported a prevalence of *H. pylori* infection in 2 of 10 (2%). Chinese children from northern Taiwan showed the presence of infection in 9 of 22 (41%) children. The response to the eradication therapy was not uniform [101, 102]. *H. pylori* has been implicated in the pathogenesis of several autoimmune diseases [90, 95, 97]. ITP is a typical organ-specific autoimmune disease. In adult patients with ITP associated to *H. pylori* infection, eradication therapy has been associated to an increase in platelet count. The Maastricht Consensus in Florence in 2012 approved, in adults with ITP and *H. pylori* infection, a similar approach to the one used in those with IDA associated to *H. pylori* infection. In the pediatric age group with cITP, diagnosis tests for identification of *H. pylori* infection, such as $^{13}$C-urea breath test, stool antigen test, or IgG serology, are not recommended. According to the guidelines described by Peter Mafertheiner, the recommendation for *H. pylori* eradication therapy in diseases like idiopathic thrombocytopenia was approved for adults [49].

Several mechanisms by which *H. pylori* may be associated to ITP have been proposed.

### 6.1. Possible mechanisms by which *H. pylori* may be related to ITP

#### *6.1.1. Molecular mimicry*

One theory is that cross-reactive antibodies produce reactions with *H. pylori* components and platelet glycoprotein through a molecular mimicry [90, 98]. Michael et al. tested platelet eluates derived from *H. pylori*-infected patients and found that platelet eluates with the capacity to react with GPIIb/IIIa or GPIb failed to recognize any *H. pylori* antigens [90]. Recently, it was reported that monoclonal antibodies generated against *H. pylori* urease B react with GPIIb/IIIa, on platelet surface, suggesting that cross-reacting antibodies may be present in ITP patients [90].

#### *6.1.2. Binding between H. pylori to von Willebrand factor/induction of platelet aggregation and apoptosis*

Many diseases associated to platelet aggregation have been described as related to *H. pylori* infection [90, 101, 103]. Myocardial infarction, coronary heart disease, and stroke are examples of this prothrombotic condition. *H. pylori* may trigger both thrombotic thrombocytopenic purpura (TTP) and ITP by the induction of the interaction among platelets and von Willebrand factor (vWF). Studies suggested that vWF is essential for platelet aggregation induced by *H. pylori* [90, 103]. The mechanisms that lead to platelet aggregation in this infection are well not understood. Byrne et al. revealed that not all *H. pylori* strains can promote platelet aggregation [96]. *H. pylori* strain 60190 (ATCC49503) induces platelet aggregation through interaction between *H. pylori*, its antibody, platelet receptor FcγRIIA (CD32), and vWF and its glycoprotein receptor (GP)Ib/IX, produced in endothelium and in megakaryocytes ($\alpha$2 granules) [103]. *H. pylori* virulence factors, the Cag pathogenicity island (CagA), and the VacA are responsible for ITP, but are not related as a cause of platelet aggregation. Platelet apoptosis has also been described. *H. pylori* promotes platelet aggregates and platelet apoptosis, which may explain the decrease in platelet counts in TTP and ITP cases [101, 103]. This may also explain the remission observed with the eradication therapy in adults. In childhood, contradictory findings with discrepancy in the response to eradication therapy suggest that in most pediatric cases ITP is primary, not secondary to *H. pylori* infection [16, 89].

#### *6.1.3. Modulation in the monocyte/macrophage function*

Change in the balance of the Fcγ receptor, related to the activation of monocytes, leads to increased monocyte function with phagocytosis and autoreactivity of B and T lymphocytes [16]. *H. pylori* can be linked to autoantibodies produced by B lymphocytes and to an over reactivation of innate and acquired immune response against platelets [16, 85, 89]. $CD4^+$ T helper cells regulate B cells, which release antithrombocyte antibodies [92, 95]. An upregulation of the genes involved in cell-related toxicity (granzime, perforin) (CD3+ CD8+ T cell) is observed [92, 104].

#### *6.1.4. Non-specific activation of immune system*

The major antigenic component for antibody production against *H. pylori* is urease. Urease antibodies initiate autoimmune responses through autoantibodies produced by the activation of B1 cells [102].

### 6.2. Genetic characteristics of the patients

Recently, the role of genetic factors has emerged, indicating that *H. pylori* patients have a lower frequency of DRB1*03 and a higher frequency of DRB1*11, DRB1*14, and DQB1*03 compared to *H. pylori*-negative patients [1, 10, 90, 101].

Based on the previously mentioned studies and mechanisms described, which lead to ITP in *H. pylori* patients, as well as the discrepancy in the response to the triple therapy in pediatric cases, to treat or not to treat *H. pylori*-infected children continues to be an unsolved question [5, 49-51].

## 7. MALT lymphoma

For the first time, in 1983, Isaacson and Wright introduced the concept of mucosa-associated lymphoid tissue (MALT), a marginal, extranodal, indolent B-cell non-Hodgkin lymphoma [105, 106]. Predominantly found in females over the age of 50, it is quite rare in childhood. In prospective, multicenter NHL-BFM treatment studies performed since 1986, composed of 2703 children, only in 4 (0.1%) MALT lymphoma was found. *H. pylori* infection was documented in two out of four of these patients [106, 107]. The clinical pathological manifestation of extranodal B cell lymphoma is similar to that presented in the MALT. MALT is a system composed of small concentrations of lymphoid tissue, containing about half the lymphocytes of the immune system [106]. Situated along the surfaces of all mucosa tissues, its principal function is to produce IgA against specific antigens on the mucosal surfaces, TH2-dependent reactions, and TH1 cytotoxic T-cell–mediated reactions, thus resulting in immune tolerance. Gut-associated lymphoid tissue (GALT), nasopharynx lymphoid tissue (NALT), and bronchus-lymphoid tissue are the most well-known examples. Also described are conjunctiva-associated lymphoid tissue (CALT), lacrimal duct–associated lymphoid tissue (LDALT), larynx-associated lymphoid tissue (LALT), and salivary duct–associated lymphoid tissue (DALT) [105-109]. Although MALT sites are separate, they are functionally connected in what is known as the "common mucosal immune system". In other words, the antigen presentation and B-cell activation at one site can result in IgA secretion at another site in a different organ. MALT tissue contains B and T cells, as well as plasma cells and macrophages. The B-cell component (MALT) is found in Peyer's patches, plasma cells of the lamina propria, and in the B-cell compartment of the mesenteric ganglia. Gastric MALT lymphoma is a clear example of lymphoid malignancy associated to chronic inflammation [105]. It can occur in the context of chronic inflammation caused by some infectious agents, such as *H. pylori* (gastric lymphoma), *Chlamydia psitacii* (ocular adnexal lymphoma), and *Borrelia burgdorferi* (cutaneous lymphoma) [105]. MALT lymphomas arise in extranodal sites, frequently found in the stomach, lungs, ocular adnexa, and thyroid as well as a small percentage in the small intestine [105, 108, 110]. In 1991, Wotherspoon et al. demonstrated, for the first time, that primary gastric lymphoma was associated to *H. pylori* infection. Later, in 1993, the same author documented regression of low-grade B-cell gastric lymphoma of MALT in five of six *H. pylori*-infected patients after eradication [9, 110, 111]. Two types of MALT lymphoma have been identified: "native MALT type" corresponding to lymphoid tissue present in the gut and "acquired MALT type" developed in response to infectious events, such as *H. pylori* infection or autoimmune diseases (Sjogren's syndrome or Hashimoto thyroiditis). The histological feature of MALT lymphoma is an infiltration of the marginal zone and diffusion into surrounding tissues, as well as the presence of lymphoepithelial lesions formed by lymphoma cells in individual mucosal glands or epithelial structures. MALT lymphoma cells have the same cytological and immunophenotype features (CD20+, CD21+ CD35+, IgM+, and IgD−) found in marginal zone B cells. Although gastric MALT lymphoma has an indolent course, rarely it can progress to aggressive high-grade tumors (extra-nodal large B cell lymphoma—eDLBCL) and, consequently, a drop in the survival rate from 90 to 40 %, respectively [105].

### 7.1. Pathogenesis and *H. pylori*

Gastric MALT lymphoma results from a multistage process that begins with the *H. pylori* infection and consequent recruitment of B and T cells [105, 112, 113]. The decrease in gastric acidity caused by the urease secretion triggers the lymphocyte infiltration and thus the establishment of MALT. B-cells are stimulated by *H. pylori* T-specific cells, acquires genetic abnormalities forming clones, possibly by trisomy 3, becoming *H. pylori*-dependent low-grade lymphoma [112, 114]. It has been demonstrated that lymphatic follicles, normally absent in the gastric mucosa, can appear, and consequently, configure the MALT after an inflammatory process [47]. *H. pylori* virulence factors seem to be crucial for the development of gastric lymphoma. CagA-positive strains are frequently related to a more aggressive lymphoma (eDLBCL) [115]. *H. pylori* can translocate the CagA protein into B-cells, inducing extracellular signal-regulated kinase activation and promoting upregulation of Bcl-2 expression, resulting in the inhibition of apoptosis. Otherwise, *H. pylori* can induce genetic mutation leading to the transformation of a normal B-cell to a malignant clone. The most frequent genetic mutations detected are t(11;18)(q21;q21), t(1;14)(p22;q32), and t(14;18)(q32;q21) involved in the activation of nuclear factor-κB (NF-κB), which plays a role in immunity, inflammation, and apoptosis [47, 113]. It has been found that positive CagA strains were higher in patients with t(11;18)(q21;q21) compared to those without such translocation (93.3 vs. 51%; P=0.01) [47, 114]. The transformation of low grade to high-grade lymphoma is rare in children, but it is documented in adults [107]. Normally, MALT lymphoma is a very indolent disease, localized for long periods of time. Systemic dissemination occurs in a few cases. In a large multicenter study of 93 patients with low-grade gastric MALT lymphoma in southern Switzerland and northern Italy, 49 *H. pylori*-infected patients with stage I of the disease. Eradication therapy was given in 97% of patients, and histological regression of MALT lymphoma was acquired in 67% of patients [114, 115]. The median time to achieve histological regression was 5 months (range 3–18 months). International guidelines recommend *H. pylori* eradication therapy in MALT lymphoma [5, 49, 50].

## 8. Diagnostic tests for *H. pylori*

Published consensus developed guidelines for the management of *H. pylori* infection in children. In 2000, ESPGHAN, and after NASPGHAN, published recommendations for *H. pylori* infection treatment [49, 51]. In 2004, the Canadian Helicobacter Study Group included consensus about how to approach *H. pylori* infection in children [5].

About testing *H. pylori* infection, questions must be asked in this age group:

Who should be tested? What tests should be used? Testing for *H. pylori* should be performed if a positive result is expected. A test and treat strategy is not recommended in children. The methods of diagnostic tests for *H. pylori* infection may be divided into two categories: invasive and non-invasive tests [5, 49-51].

### 8.1. Invasive tests

Invasive tests require a gastric endoscopy and a biopsy with culture for detecting *H. pylori* [116, 117]. They are the only tests considered to be 100% specific. The hematoxylin–eosin (HE) stain usually shows *H. pylori* strains [114, 118]. Nevertheless, when the results are inconclusive, there are at least two different stain techniques to be used on biopsied tissue: HE to evaluate inflammatory cells and Giemsa or Genta stain to detect *H. pylori*. Although the Genta stain due to a combination between a silver stain, HE and Alcian blue can visualize both inflammatory cells and *H. pylori* strain with higher accuracy, this formulation is technically complex. In contrast, the Giemsa stain is technically simple, highly sensitive, and inexpensive [117, 119].

#### *8.1.1. Rapid urease test (RUT)*

RUT identifies *H. pylori* through urease activity of the bacteria in gastric mucosa [120, 121]. Gastric biopsies are obtained and placed into an agar gel on a reaction contained urea, a buffer, and a pH-sensitive indicator. In presence of *H. pylori*, urea is metabolized to ammonia and bicarbonate leading to an increase of gastric pH, with changing in color [8, 117, 118]. The low cost, the simplicity, and rapid results make this test practical and effective, as long as the patient has not taken proton pump inhibitors or antibiotics. Medication that reduces the density of bacteria can decrease the sensitivity of the RUT up to 25%. Therefore, proton pumps and antibiotics must be not taken 1–2 weeks before the procedure [5, 49-51]..

#### *8.1.2. Histology*

Histology is considered a standard method for detecting *H. pylori* infection. The sensitivity and specificity vary according to the site, number, and size of the biopsies, and also the experience of the pathologist [82, 117, 118]. False results can be obtained with a low density of bacteria. In these cases, multiple biopsies are needed. The majority of gastroenterologists obtained only biopsies of the antrum [122]. Recent studies revealed that the addition of corpus biopsies to antral biopsies increase the probability of *H. pylori* identification in all infected patients [50, 51, 117, 118].

#### *8.1.3. Cultures*

Cultures method has high specificity for the diagnosis of *H. pylori* infection, normally unnecessary for routine the diagnosis of *H. pylori*. The principal indication is testing for antimicrobial sensitivity in order to choose the appropriate antibiotic. Cultures are expensive and not as sensitive as RUT or histology and not available in many clinical laboratories [119, 120].

*8.1.4. Polymerase chain reaction*

PCR is a DNA amplification that uses the rapid production of a target DNA sequence to identify *H. pylori*. It is capable of identifying *H. pylori* strains in biopsies with chronic gastritis and non-identifiable bacteria. PCR can be performed on samples obtained by invasive and non-invasive methods using samples obtained of saliva, gastric juice, and stools [82, 119]. It is simple to perform and can provide additional genotypic information about the strain and antibiotic susceptibilities. PCR could be complete in 3–4 hours, and it is capable to detect the point mutations attributed to the development of clarithromycin resistance [119, 123].

### 8.2. Non-invasive tests

Although the gold standard method for diagnosis is gastric histology and rapid urea test, an important disadvantage is their invasiveness. Non-invasive tests, such as urea breath test (UBT), serology, and more recently, fecal *H. pylori* antigen, have been developed and all of them are feasible in children [50, 119].

*8.2.1. Urea breath test (UBT)*

UBT is one of the preferred tests to diagnose active *H. pylori* infection [5, 124]. It is based on hydrolyses of urea to ammonia and carbon dioxide, which diffuses into the blood and is excreted by the lungs. Since it requires the child's full cooperation, it is difficult to perform in children, especially toddlers and physically challenged [50]. This test is based on the ingestion of urea labeled with either non-radioactive isotype ($C^{13}$) or radioactive isotype ($C^{12}$). The first is preferred in children [5]. Labeled urea is dissolved in orange juice without sugar, given in fasting, and the primary objective is to validate $C^{13}$ in children and adolescents. The ratio in exhaled air is measured at 0 and then 30 minutes after the intake, and the test is considered positive when the difference between these two ratios exceeds 4‰ (cut-off value) [124]. Antibiotics must be withheld at least 28 days and proton pump inhibitor (PPI) for 7–14 days before UBT [5, 82, 124].

*8.2.2. Antibody test*

The IgG-specific *H. pylori* antibodies are present in blood nearly 21 days after the infection and can persist for a long time after eradication therapy. With a sensitivity of 85% and specificity of 79%, they are not adequate for documenting *H. pylori* eradication [6, 50].

*8.2.3. Fecal antigen test*

The fecal antigen test (FAT) identifies *H. pylori* in stool by enzyme immunoassay (EIA) based on polyclonal or monoclonal antibodies, and immunochromatographic tests, so-called rapid or quick tests. The first commercial EIA test to detect *H. pylori* antigen in stool was the Premier Platinum HpSA based on polyclonal antibodies. These tests have a wide range of sensitivity and specificity both in pretreatment (86, 90–98%) and post-treatment (89, 91–92, 95%) [51]. The stool antigen tests using polyclonal antibodies demonstrated variable results and seem to have less accuracy than those using monoclonal antibodies. This diagnostic approach is convenient for children in whom it is easy to collect feces [117]. Nguyen et al. evaluated the sensitivity and specificity of monoclonal enzyme stool antigen assay for diagnosis of *H. pylori* in 232 children age range 3–5 years *H. pylori* infection positive by culture from biopsies. They found a sensitivity of 96% and a specificity of 94.8% [125, 126]. FAT can be used to screen for infection before and after treatment [50, 82, 117]. It is considered as acceptable as UBT and is not dependent on the child′s collaboration. Recent studies indicate that FAT can be done as early as 14 days after treatment, but should be done more than 4 weeks [50].

Note: PPI must be withheld two weeks before performing RUT, UBT, and FAT [49, 51]

## 9. Treatment

The goal of treatment is to obtain 90% eradication. The therapeutic regimens are variable and dependent on local resistance data. Several studies have documented high resistance to clarithromycin and metronidazole [127]. The first treatment commonly administered in children and adults is a triple therapy, for 14 days, that includes a PPI and two antibiotics, amoxicillin and metronidazole or clarithromycin [49-51, 127]. The first line of recommended eradication therapies are as follows: amoxicillin, 50 mg/kg twice a day for 14 days; clarithromycin, 15 mg/kg/twice daily for 14 days; and PPI, 1 mg/kg twice daily for 1 month. Alternatively, amoxicillin, 50 mg/kg twice a day for 14 days; metronidazole, 20 mg/kg twice daily for 14 days; and PPI, 1 mg/kg twice daily for 1 month or clarithromycin, 15 mg/kg/twice daily for 14 days; metronidazole, 20 mg/kg twice daily for 14 days; and PPI, 1 mg/kg twice daily for 1 month [50]. Several studies revealed that the use of probiotics improves the treatment tolerance, but there is no evidence of higher eradication [82]. Koletzko et al. [122] revealed a rate of resistance to clarithromycin of 20%, and a rate of resistance to metronidazole of 23% after a first treatment [82, 127]. In Portugal, a higher clarithromycin resistance rate was reported in children (44.8%) compared with adults (14.8%) [127]. The main factors for triple therapy failure are the low compliance and the bacteria's resistance to antibiotics. The risk for clarithromycin resistance is related with the previous consumption of macrolides, which is substantially prescribed in children for respiratory tract diseases. Double resistance strains were found in up to 50% of strains after failure of therapy using both clarithromycin and metronidazole [128]. The failure after the first therapeutic approach is predictive of resistance to other therapeutic approaches [50, 51, 128]. NASPHGAN recommend, in case of failure in the first line of treatment in children, and if possible, to perform culture with testing for antibiotic sensitivity to guide a second-line therapy. Other options may be taken if a *H. pylori* culture is not possible: quadruple therapy composed of PPI + metronidazole + amoxicillin + bismuth, triple therapy using fluoroquinolones, but of limited indication in children, or sequential therapy involving dual therapy with PPI and amoxicillin for 5 days followed sequentially by 5 days of triple therapy with PPI, clarithromycin, and metronidazole/tinidazole. In 2005, 74 children (randomized) received sequential therapy and triple therapy. Eradication was 97.3% in those with sequential therapy compared with 75.7% in children with triple therapy [51].

## 10. Conclusion and possibilities of new studies

Approximately 50% of the world's population is *H. pylori* infected. Although it has been a part of human microbiota, it is classified by The World Health Organization as a gastric carcinogenic. *H. pylori* is acquired essentially in childhood and through mechanisms of escape, it persists in gastric mucosa for life if left untreated. An association has been found between *H. pylori* infection and poverty, low socioeconomic conditions, poor hygiene, and nutritional deficiencies. With higher prevalence in developing countries, the predisposing factors are the high number of residents in the same home, sharing the same room or the same bed with *H. pylori*-infected children, as well as poor sanitary conditions. Hematological extragastric disorders have been described as being associated to *H. pylori* infection. Unexplained ID, IDA, and refractory IDA in childhood are the most well-known pathologies related to *H. pylori* infection. Two meta-analysis have supported the association between *H. pylori* infection and IDA, showing an increase of hemoglobin levels after *H. pylori* eradication [10, 45]. Many areas of the world have high prevalence of both *H. pylori* infection and IDA. ID in children leads to major consequences on children's health and neurodevelopment. Associations have been reported, in children, between IDA, lower intelligence scores or cognitive functioning in tests, and behavioral delays in children, showing that treatment can improve these outcomes [127, 129]. As a result, Update of US Preventive Services Task Force (USPSTF) and the Center for Disease Control and Prevention recommend screening for IDA in children aged 6–24 months, between 9 and 12 months, 6 months later, and then annually from the ages of 2 to 5 years, respectively, and to treat the ID by prescribing 3 mg/kg/day of iron drops between feedings [129-131]. Refractory to iron therapy implies, after the exclusion of ingestion deficiencies, hemorrhage, absorption problems, and (rarely) metabolic abnormalities, the search for *H. pylori* infection using in the first line non-invasive tests (UBT, FAT, and specific IgG *H. pylori* antibodies). All non-invasive tests are feasible in clinical use. $C^{13}$UBT, with a good sensitivity for the diagnosis of *H. pylori* infection, shows limitations such as low specificity for very young children, being affected by previous ingestion of antibiotics or PPI and the requirement of patient cooperation [49-51]. Stool antigen test shows low sensitivity and good specificity in children of all ages, limited also by PPI and antibiotics. It is advisable to validate two non-invasive tests, the $C^{13}$UBT and stool antigen for the diagnosis of *H. pylori* infection in pediatric ages. Serology is based on the immunological response to chronic *H. pylori* gastric inflammation and is not dependent on antibiotics or on the loading of gastric bacteria. International Guidelines are well defined regarding IDA in the context of *H. pylori* infection in childhood, in which eradication therapy is indicated as it is done in adults. Consensus about the approach of cTPI and *H. pylori* infection is well defined in adults, in which *H. pylori* eradication is followed by platelet recuperation. In childhood, there is no evidence to support a relationship between this infection and cTPI. Reports about prevalence of *H. pylori* and TPI seem to be according to the epidemiological data of the countries. Contradictory findings with discrepancy in the response to eradication therapy suggest that in most pediatric cases ITP is primary, with a spontaneous cure from 6 months to 1 year later, and not secondary to *H. pylori* infection [87-89]. Maastricht IV and other guidelines suggest not searching for or treating *H. pylori* in this context.

Gastric MALT lymphoma is a lymphoid malignancy that is quite rare in children. In these cases, eradication therapy must be performed regardless of the stage of lymphoma. The failure of *H. pylori* eradication is predictive of a resistant strain acquisition and also predictive of subsequent therapeutic failure. A primary *H. pylori* resistance in children of European countries has been estimated and ranges from 12.45 to 23.5% [128]. Therefore, clarithromycin-based triple therapy can be recommended after studies of antibiotic susceptibility or in countries with low resistance to clarithromycin. The high resistance of *H. pylori* to clarithromycin can justify the use, as first-line therapeutic approach in children, of the sequential therapy which was referred, resulting in eradication rates of 97.3% against 75.7% with triple therapy [49, 51]. In children, there are particular problems with alternative antibiotics, which are not approved for the age. Therefore, they are often treated multiple times without cure. The impact of this infection on public health implies applying active measures toward H. pylori eradication. A vaccination strategy should be implemented as the best option to eliminate H. pylori and therefore to improve public health.

## 11. New studies

Several new antibiotics are under investigation for the treatment of H. pylori in adults. (1) Rifabutin. Triple therapy for 10 days with rifabutin + pantoprazole + amoxicillin is showing good results in resistant H. pylori areas. Resulting in eradication rates of 50% [82, 132]; (2) Nitazoxanide that includes levofloxacin, nitazoxanide, doxycycline, and omeprazole is showing better efficacy than standard triple therapy [133].

## Author details

Natalina Miguel*

Address all correspondence to: natalina.miguel@gmail.com

Pediatric Department -Trás-os-Montes e Alto-Douro Hospital Center, Vila Real, Portugal

The author has no conflict of interest.

## References

[1] Papagiannakis P, Michalopoulos C, Papalexi F, Dalampoura D, Diamantidis MD. The role of Helicobacter pylori infection in hematological disorders. Eur J Intern Med. 2013 Dec;24(8):685-90. PubMed PMID: 23523153. Epub 2013/03/26. eng.

[2] Marshall BJ, Warren JR. Unidentified curved bacilli in the stomach of patients with gastritis and peptic ulceration. Lancet. 1984 Jun 16;1(8390):1311-5. PubMed PMID: 6145023. Epub 1984/06/16. eng.

[3] Cardenas VM, Mulla ZD, Ortiz M, Graham DY. Iron deficiency and Helicobacter pylori infection in the United States. Am J Epidemiol. 2006 Jan 15;163(2):127-34. PubMed PMID: 16306309. Epub 2005/11/25. eng.

[4] Rajindrajith S, Devanarayana NM, de Silva HJ. Helicobacter pylori infection in children. Saudi J Gastroenterol. 2009 Apr;15(2):86-94. PubMed PMID: 19568571. Pubmed Central PMCID: PMC2702974. Epub 2009/07/02. eng.

[5] Sherman P, Hassall E, Hunt RH, Fallone CA, Veldhuyzen Van Zanten S, Thomson AB. Canadian Helicobacter Study Group Consensus Conference on the Approach to Helicobacter pylori Infection in Children and Adolescents. Can J Gastroenterol. 1999 Sep;13(7):553-9. PubMed PMID: 10519952. Epub 1999/10/16. eng.

[6] Schistosomes, liver flukes and Helicobacter pylori. IARC Working Group on the Evaluation of Carcinogenic Risks to Humans. Lyon, 7-14 June 1994. IARC Monogr Eval Carcinog Risks Hum. 1994;61:1-241. PubMed PMID: 7715068. Epub 1994/01/01. eng.

[7] Blaser MJ. Who are we? Indigenous microbes and the ecology of human diseases. EMBO Rep. 2006 Oct;7(10):956-60. PubMed PMID: 17016449. Pubmed Central PMCID: PMC1618379. Epub 2006/10/04. eng.

[8] Kusters JG, van Vliet AH, Kuipers EJ. Pathogenesis of Helicobacter pylori infection. Clin Microbiol Rev. 2006 Jul;19(3):449-90. PubMed PMID: 16847081. Pubmed Central PMCID: PMC1539101. Epub 2006/07/19. eng.

[9] Wotherspoon AC, Ortiz-Hidalgo C, Falzon MR, Isaacson PG. Helicobacter pylori-associated gastritis and primary B-cell gastric lymphoma. Lancet. 1991 Nov 9;338(8776): 1175-6. PubMed PMID: 1682595. Epub 1991/11/09. eng.

[10] Pacifico L, Osborn JF, Tromba V, Romaggioli S, Bascetta S, Chiesa C. Helicobacter pylori infection and extragastric disorders in children: a critical update. World J Gastroenterol. 2014 Feb 14;20(6):1379-401. PubMed PMID: 24587617. Pubmed Central PMCID: PMC3925850. Epub 2014/03/04. eng.

[11] Hershko C, Ronson A, Souroujon M, Maschler I, Heyd J, Patz J. Variable hematologic presentation of autoimmune gastritis: age-related progression from iron deficiency to cobalamin depletion. Blood. 2006 Feb 15;107(4):1673-9. PubMed PMID: 16239424. Epub 2005/10/22. eng.

[12] Hershko C, Hoffbrand AV, Keret D, Souroujon M, Maschler I, Monselise Y, et al. Role of autoimmune gastritis, Helicobacter pylori and celiac disease in refractory or unexplained iron deficiency anemia. Haematologica. 2005 May;90(5):585-95. PubMed PMID: 15921373. Epub 2005/06/01. eng.

[13] Hershko C, Camaschella C. How I treat unexplained refractory iron deficiency anemia. Blood. 2014 Jan 16;123(3):326-33. PubMed PMID: 24215034. Epub 2013/11/12. eng.

[14] Smyk DS, Koutsoumpas AL, Mytilinaiou MG, Rigopoulou EI, Sakkas LI, Bogdanos DP. Helicobacter pylori and autoimmune disease: cause or bystander. World J Gastroenterol. 2014 Jan 21;20(3):613-29. PubMed PMID: 24574735. Pubmed Central PMCID: PMC3921471. Epub 2014/02/28. eng.

[15] Ertem D. Helicobacter pylori infection in children. Journal of Pediatric Sciences. 2011;3(4)(e 102):1-15.

[16] Campuzano-Maya G. Hematologic manifestations of Helicobacter pylori infection. World J Gastroenterol. 2014 Sep 28;20(36):12818-38. PubMed PMID: 25278680. Pubmed Central PMCID: PMC4177465. Epub 2014/10/04. eng.

[17] Smith SM. Role of Toll-like receptors in Helicobacter pylori infection and immunity. World J Gastrointest Pathophysiol. 2014 Aug 15;5(3):133-46. PubMed PMID: 25133016. Pubmed Central PMCID: PMC4133513. Epub 2014/08/19. eng.

[18] Smith SM, Moran AP, Duggan SP, Ahmed SE, Mohamed AS, Windle HJ, et al. Tribbles 3: a novel regulator of TLR2-mediated signaling in response to Helicobacter pylori lipopolysaccharide. J Immunol. 2011 Feb 15;186(4):2462-71. PubMed PMID: 21220698. Epub 2011/01/12. eng.

[19] Michalkiewicz J, Helmin-Basa A, Grzywa R, Czerwionka-Szaflarska M, Szaflarska-Poplawska A, Mierzwa G, et al. Innate immunity components and cytokines in gastric mucosa in children with Helicobacter pylori infection. Mediators Inflamm. 2015;2015:176726. PubMed PMID: 25948881. Pubmed Central PMCID: PMC4407632. Epub 2015/05/08. eng.

[20] Mogensen TH. Pathogen recognition and inflammatory signaling in innate immune defenses. Clin Microbiol Rev. 2009 Apr;22(2):240-73, Table of Contents. PubMed PMID: 19366914. Pubmed Central PMCID: Pmc2668232. Epub 2009/04/16. eng.

[21] Peek RM, Jr., Fiske C, Wilson KT. Role of innate immunity in Helicobacter pylori-induced gastric malignancy. Physiol Rev. 2010 Jul;90(3):831-58. PubMed PMID: 20664074. Pubmed Central PMCID: Pmc2990353. Epub 2010/07/29. eng.

[22] Wang JQ, Jeelall YS, Ferguson LL, Horikawa K. Toll-Like Receptors and Cancer: MYD88 Mutation and Inflammation. Front Immunol. 2014;5:367. PubMed PMID: 25132836. Pubmed Central PMCID: PMC4116802. Epub 2014/08/19. eng.

[23] Bliss CM, Jr., Golenbock DT, Keates S, Linevsky JK, Kelly CP. Helicobacter pylori lipopolysaccharide binds to CD14 and stimulates release of interleukin-8, epithelial neutrophil-activating peptide 78, and monocyte chemotactic protein 1 by human monocytes. Infect Immun. 1998 Nov;66(11):5357-63. PubMed PMID: 9784544. Pubmed Central PMCID: PMC108670. Epub 1998/10/24. eng.

[24] Ford JW, McVicar DW. TREM and TREM-like receptors in inflammation and disease. Curr Opin Immunol. 2009 Feb;21(1):38-46. PubMed PMID: 19230638. Pubmed Central PMCID: Pmc2723941. Epub 2009/02/24. eng.

[25] Roe K, Gibot S, Verma S. Triggering receptor expressed on myeloid cells-1 (TREM-1): a new player in antiviral immunity? Front Microbiol. 2014;5:627. PubMed PMID: 25505454. Pubmed Central PMCID: Pmc4244588. Epub 2014/12/17. eng.

[26] Schmausser B, Endrich S, Beier D, Moran AP, Burek CJ, Rosenwald A, et al. Triggering receptor expressed on myeloid cells-1 (TREM-1) expression on gastric epithelium: implication for a role of TREM-1 in Helicobacter pylori infection. Clin Exp Immunol. 2008 Apr;152(1):88-94. PubMed PMID: 18321350. Pubmed Central PMCID: Pmc2384064. Epub 2008/03/07. eng.

[27] Amedei A, Cappon A, Codolo G, Cabrelle A, Polenghi A, Benagiano M, et al. The neutrophil-activating protein of Helicobacter pylori promotes Th1 immune responses. J Clin Invest. 2006 Apr;116(4):1092-101. PubMed PMID: 16543949. Pubmed Central PMCID: PMC1401483. Epub 2006/03/18. eng.

[28] Larussa T, Leone I, Suraci E, Imeneo M, Luzza F. Helicobacter pylori and T Helper Cells: Mechanisms of Immune Escape and Tolerance. J Immunol Res. 2015;2015:981328. PubMed PMID: 26525279. Pubmed Central PMCID: PMC4615206. Epub 2015/11/04. eng.

[29] Everhart JE, Kruszon-Moran D, Perez-Perez GI, Tralka TS, McQuillan G. Seroprevalence and ethnic differences in Helicobacter pylori infection among adults in the United States. J Infect Dis. 2000 Apr;181(4):1359-63. PubMed PMID: 10762567. Epub 2000/04/14. eng.

[30] Franceschi F, Annalisa T, Teresa DR, Giovanna D, Ianiro G, Franco S, et al. Role of Helicobacter pylori infection on nutrition and metabolism. World J Gastroenterol. 2014 Sep 28;20(36):12809-17. PubMed PMID: 25278679. Pubmed Central PMCID: Pmc4177464. Epub 2014/10/04. eng.

[31] Nguyen VB, Nguyen TAX, Nguyen TVA, PHAM DP, Hoang TH, Phung DC. Epidemiology of helicobacter pylori infection in Kinh and Khmer Children in Mekong Delta, Vietnam. Ann Clin Lab Res. 2015:1-9.

[32] Mitchel H. Epidemiology of Infection. In: HLT M, GL M, SL H, editors. Helicobacter pylori: Physiology and Genetics: Washington (DC): ASM Press; 2001.

[33] Cherian S, Forbes D, Sanfilippo F, Cook A, Burgner D. The epidemiology of Helicobacter pylori infection in African refugee children resettled in Australia. Med J Aust. 2008 Oct 20;189(8):438-41. PubMed PMID: 18928436. Epub 2008/10/22. eng.

[34] Brown LM. Helicobacter pylori: epidemiology and routes of transmission. Epidemiol Rev. 2000;22(2):283-97. PubMed PMID: 11218379. Epub 2001/02/24. eng.

[35] Goodman KJ, Correa P, Tengana Aux HJ, DeLany JP, Collazos T. Nutritional factors and Helicobacter pylori infection in Colombian children. J Pediatr Gastroenterol Nutr. 1997 Nov;25(5):507-15. PubMed PMID: 9360204. Epub 1997/11/14. eng.

[36] Reibman J, Marmor M, Filner J, Fernandez-Beros ME, Rogers L, Perez-Perez GI, et al. Asthma is inversely associated with Helicobacter pylori status in an urban population. PLoS One. 2008;3(12):e4060. PubMed PMID: 19112508. Pubmed Central PMCID: PMC2603593. Epub 2008/12/30. eng.

[37] Amedei A, Codolo G, Del Prete G, de Bernard M, D'Elios MM. The effect of Helicobacter pylori on asthma and allergy. J Asthma Allergy. 2010;3:139-47. PubMed PMID: 21437048. Pubmed Central PMCID: Pmc3047919. Epub 2010/01/01. eng.

[38] Farinha P, Gascoyne RD. Helicobacter pylori and MALT lymphoma. Gastroenterology. 2005 May;128(6):1579-605. PubMed PMID: 15887153. Epub 2005/05/12. eng.

[39] Hulten K, Han SW, Enroth H, Klein PD, Opekun AR, Gilman RH, et al. Helicobacter pylori in the drinking water in Peru. Gastroenterology. 1996 Apr;110(4):1031-5. PubMed PMID: 8612990. Epub 1996/04/01. eng.

[40] Fan XG, Chua A, Li TG, Zeng QS. Survival of Helicobacter pylori in milk and tap water. J Gastroenterol Hepatol. 1998 Nov;13(11):1096-8. PubMed PMID: 9870794. Epub 1998/12/31. eng.

[41] Parsonnet J, Shmuely H, Haggerty T. Fecal and oral shedding of Helicobacter pylori from healthy infected adults. JAMA. 1999 Dec 15;282(23):2240-5. PubMed PMID: 10605976. Epub 1999/12/22. eng.

[42] Ferguson DA, Jr., Li C, Patel NR, Mayberry WR, Chi DS, Thomas E. Isolation of Helicobacter pylori from saliva. J Clin Microbiol. 1993 Oct;31(10):2802-4. PubMed PMID: 8253990. Pubmed Central PMCID: Pmc266021. Epub 1993/10/01. eng.

[43] Handt LK, Fox JG, Dewhirst FE, Fraser GJ, Paster BJ, Yan LL, et al. Helicobacter pylori isolated from the domestic cat: public health implications. Infect Immun. 1994 Jun; 62(6):2367-74. PubMed PMID: 8188360. Pubmed Central PMCID: Pmc186520. Epub 1994/06/01. eng.

[44] Roesler BM, Rabelo-Goncalves EM, Zeitune JM. Virulence Factors of Helicobacter pylori: A Review. Clin Med Insights Gastroenterol. 2014;7:9-17. PubMed PMID: 24833944. Pubmed Central PMCID: PMC4019226. Epub 2014/05/17. eng.

[45] Pacifico L, Anania C, Osborn JF, Ferraro F, Chiesa C. Consequences of Helicobacter pylori infection in children. World J Gastroenterol. 2010 Nov 7;16(41):5181-94. PubMed PMID: 21049552. Pubmed Central PMCID: Pmc2975089. Epub 2010/11/05. eng.

[46] Rogers LM, Boy E, Miller JW, Green R, Rodriguez M, Chew F, et al. Predictors of cobalamin deficiency in Guatemalan school children: diet, Helicobacter pylori, or bacte-

rial overgrowth? J Pediatr Gastroenterol Nutr. 2003 Jan;36(1):27-36. PubMed PMID: 12499993. Epub 2002/12/25. eng.

[47] Zullo A, Hassan C, Ridola L, Repici A, Manta R, Andriani A. Gastric MALT lymphoma: old and new insights. Ann Gastroenterol. 2014;27(1):27-33. PubMed PMID: 24714739. Pubmed Central PMCID: Pmc3959547. Epub 2014/04/10. Eng.

[48] Konturek SJ, Konturek PC, Pieniazek P, Bielanski W. Role of Helicobacter pylori infection in extragastroduodenal disorders: introductory remarks. J Physiol Pharmacol. 1999 Dec;50(5):683-94. PubMed PMID: 10695551. Epub 2000/03/01. eng.

[49] Malfertheiner P, F. M, C. OM. Guidelines for the management of Helicobacter pylori Infection. European Gastroenterol Review. 2005:59-999.

[50] Chey WD, Wong BC. American College of Gastroenterology guideline on the management of Helicobacter pylori infection. Am J Gastroenterol. 2007 Aug;102(8): 1808-25. PubMed PMID: 17608775. Epub 2007/07/05. eng.

[51] Koletzko S, Jones NL, Goodman KJ, Gold B, Rowland M, Cadranel S, et al. Evidence-based guidelines from ESPGHAN and NASPGHAN for Helicobacter pylori infection in children. J Pediatr Gastroenterol Nutr. 2011 Aug;53(2):230-43. PubMed PMID: 21558964. Epub 2011/05/12. eng.

[52] Gupta V, Eden AJ, Mills MJ. Helicobacter pylori and autoimmune neutropenia. Clin Lab Haematol. 2002 Jun;24(3):183-5. PubMed PMID: 12067285. Epub 2002/06/18. eng.

[53] Papadaki HA, Pontikoglou C, Eliopoulos DG, Pyrovolaki K, Spyridaki R, Eliopoulos GD. Helicobacter pylori infection is probably the cause of chronic idiopathic neutropenia (CIN)-associated splenomegaly. Am J Hematol. 2006 Feb;81(2):142-4. PubMed PMID: 16432851. Epub 2006/01/25. eng.

[54] Qu XH, Huang XL, Xiong P, Zhu CY, Huang YL, Lu LG, et al. Does Helicobacter pylori infection play a role in iron deficiency anemia? A meta-analysis. World J Gastroenterol. 2010 Feb 21;16(7):886-96. PubMed PMID: 20143469. Pubmed Central PMCID: PMC2825337. Epub 2010/02/10. eng.

[55] Dufour C, Brisigotti M, Fabretti G, Luxardo P, Mori PG, Barabino A. Helicobacter pylori gastric infection and sideropenic refractory anemia. J Pediatr Gastroenterol Nutr. 1993 Aug;17(2):225-7. PubMed PMID: 8229554. Epub 1993/08/01. eng.

[56] Gasbarrini A, Franceschi F, Armuzzi A, Ojetti V, Candelli M, Torre ES, et al. Extradigestive manifestations of Helicobacter pylori gastric infection. Gut. 1999 Jul;45 Suppl 1:I9-i12. PubMed PMID: 10457029. Pubmed Central PMCID: Pmc1766655. Epub 1999/08/24. eng.

[57] Kearney DJ. Helicobacter pylori infection and iron deficiency anemia: accumulating evidence in support of a real association. Indian J Gastroenterol. 2005 Jul-Aug;24(4): 147-50. PubMed PMID: 16204900. Epub 2005/10/06. eng.

[58] Jain S, Das S, Gupta P. Fecal occult blood screening in children with severe malnutrition. Indian Pediatr. 2007 Dec;44(12):913-5. PubMed PMID: 18175844. Epub 2008/01/08. eng.

[59] Bodger K, Crabtree JE. Helicobacter pylori and gastric inflammation. Br Med Bull. 1998;54(1):139-50. PubMed PMID: 9604438. Epub 1998/05/30. eng.

[60] Rieder G, Einsiedl W, Hatz RA, Stolte M, Enders GA, Walz A. Comparison of CXC chemokines ENA-78 and interleukin-8 expression in Helicobacter pylori-associated gastritis. Infect Immun. 2001 Jan;69(1):81-8. PubMed PMID: 11119492. Pubmed Central PMCID: Pmc97858. Epub 2000/12/19. eng.

[61] Verga Falzacappa MV, Vujic Spasic M, Kessler R, Stolte J, Hentze MW, Muckenthaler MU. STAT3 mediates hepatic hepcidin expression and its inflammatory stimulation. Blood. 2007 Jan 1;109(1):353-8. PubMed PMID: 16946298. Epub 2006/09/02. eng.

[62] Cherian S, Forbes DA, Cook AG, Sanfilippo FM, Kemna EH, Swinkels DW, et al. An insight into the relationships between hepcidin, anemia, infections and inflammatory cytokines in pediatric refugees: a cross-sectional study. PLoS One. 2008;3(12):e4030. PubMed PMID: 19107209. Pubmed Central PMCID: Pmc2603326. Epub 2008/12/25. eng.

[63] Andrews NC. Anemia of inflammation: the cytokine-hepcidin link. J Clin Invest. 2004 May;113(9):1251-3. PubMed PMID: 15124013. Pubmed Central PMCID: Pmc398435. Epub 2004/05/05. eng.

[64] Weinstein DA, Roy CN, Fleming MD, Loda MF, Wolfsdorf JI, Andrews NC. Inappropriate expression of hepcidin is associated with iron refractory anemia: implications for the anemia of chronic disease. Blood. 2002 Nov 15;100(10):3776-81. PubMed PMID: 12393428. Epub 2002/10/24. eng.

[65] Lee SY, Song EY, Yun YM, Yoon SY, Cho YH, Kim SY, et al. Serum prohepcidin levels in Helicobacter pylori infected patients with iron deficiency anemia. Korean J Intern Med. 2010 Jun;25(2):195-200. PubMed PMID: 20526394. Pubmed Central PMCID: Pmc2880694. Epub 2010/06/09. eng.

[66] Baysoy G, Ertem D, Ademoglu E, Kotiloglu E, Keskin S, Pehlivanoglu E. Gastric histopathology, iron status and iron deficiency anemia in children with Helicobacter pylori infection. J Pediatr Gastroenterol Nutr. 2004 Feb;38(2):146-51. PubMed PMID: 14734875. Epub 2004/01/22. eng.

[67] Przybyszewska J, Zekanowska E. The role of hepcidin, ferroportin, HCP1, and DMT1 protein in iron absorption in the human digestive tract. Prz Gastroenterol. 2014;9(4): 208-13. PubMed PMID: 25276251. Pubmed Central PMCID: Pmc4178046. Epub 2014/10/03. eng.

[68] Ganz T. Hepcidin, a key regulator of iron metabolism and mediator of anemia of inflammation. Blood. 2003 Aug 1;102(3):783-8. PubMed PMID: 12663437. Epub 2003/03/29. eng.

[69] Kim HK, Jang EC, Yeom JO, Kim SY, Cho H, Kim SS, et al. Serum prohepcidin levels are lower in patients with atrophic gastritis. Gastroenterol Res Pract.

2013;2013:201810. PubMed PMID: 23533385. Pubmed Central PMCID: Pmc3603588. Epub 2013/03/28. eng.

[70] Harris PR, Serrano CA, Villagran A, Walker MM, Thomson M, Duarte I, et al. Helicobacter pylori-associated hypochlorhydria in children, and development of iron deficiency. J Clin Pathol. 2013 Apr;66(4):343-7. PubMed PMID: 23268321. Epub 2012/12/27. eng.

[71] Sarker SA, Davidsson L, Mahmud H, Walczyk T, Hurrell RF, Gyr N, et al. Helicobacter pylori infection, iron absorption, and gastric acid secretion in Bangladeshi children. Am J Clin Nutr. 2004 Jul;80(1):149-53. PubMed PMID: 15213042. Epub 2004/06/24. eng.

[72] Modlin IM, Kidd M, Marks IN, Tang LH. The pivotal role of John S. Edkins in the discovery of gastrin. World J Surg. 1997 Feb;21(2):226-34. PubMed PMID: 8995084. Epub 1997/02/01. eng.

[73] Korman MG, Strickland RG, Hansky J. Serum gastrin in chronic gastritis. Br Med J. 1971 Apr 3;2(5752):16-8. PubMed PMID: 5550864. Pubmed Central PMCID: Pmc1795895. Epub 1971/04/03. eng.

[74] Hartman KR, Barker JA. Microcytic anemia with iron malabsorption: an inherited disorder of iron metabolism. Am J Hematol. 1996 Apr;51(4):269-75. PubMed PMID: 8602626. Epub 1996/04/01. eng.

[75] Chen LH, Luo HS. Effects of H pylori therapy on erythrocytic and iron parameters in iron deficiency anemia patients with H pylori-positive chronic gastristis. World J Gastroenterol. 2007 Oct 28;13(40):5380-3. PubMed PMID: 17879411. Pubmed Central PMCID: PMC4171331. Epub 2007/09/20. eng.

[76] Park JH, Kim SY, Kim DW, Lee WG, Rhee KH, Youn HS. Correlation between Helicobacter pylori infection and vitamin C levels in whole blood, plasma, and gastric juice, and the pH of gastric juice in Korean children. J Pediatr Gastroenterol Nutr. 2003 Jul;37(1): 53-62. PubMed PMID: 12827006. Epub 2003/06/27. eng.

[77] Zhang ZW, Patchett SE, Perrett D, Katelaris PH, Domizio P, Farthing MJ. The relation between gastric vitamin C concentrations, mucosal histology, and CagA seropositivity in the human stomach. Gut. 1998 Sep;43(3):322-6. PubMed PMID: 9863475. Pubmed Central PMCID: Pmc1727232. Epub 1998/12/24. eng.

[78] Annibale B, Marignani M, Monarca B, Antonelli G, Marcheggiano A, Martino G, et al. Reversal of iron deficiency anemia after Helicobacter pylori eradication in patients with asymptomatic gastritis. Ann Intern Med. 1999 Nov 2;131(9):668-72. PubMed PMID: 10577329. Epub 1999/11/30. eng.

[79] Zhang ZW, Abdullahi M, Farthing MJ. Effect of physiological concentrations of vitamin C on gastric cancer cells and Helicobacter pylori. Gut. 2002 Feb;50(2):165-9. PubMed PMID: 11788554. Pubmed Central PMCID: Pmc1773094. Epub 2002/01/15. eng.

[80] Annibale B, Capurso G, Lahner E, Passi S, Ricci R, Maggio F, et al. Concomitant alterations in intragastric pH and ascorbic acid concentration in patients with Helicobacter pylori gastritis and associated iron deficiency anaemia. Gut. 2003 Apr;52(4): 496-501. PubMed PMID: 12631657. Pubmed Central PMCID: PMC1773597. Epub 2003/03/13. eng.

[81] Senkovich O, Ceaser S, McGee DJ, Testerman TL. Unique host iron utilization mechanisms of Helicobacter pylori revealed with iron-deficient chemically defined media. Infect Immun. 2010 May;78(5):1841-9. PubMed PMID: 20176792. Pubmed Central PMCID: Pmc2863533. Epub 2010/02/24. eng.

[82] Testerman TL, Morris J. Beyond the stomach: an updated view of Helicobacter pylori pathogenesis, diagnosis, and treatment. World J Gastroenterol. 2014 Sep 28;20(36): 12781-808. PubMed PMID: 25278678. Pubmed Central PMCID: Pmc4177463. Epub 2014/10/04. eng.

[83] Dogan Y, Erkan T, Onal Z, Usta M, Dogusoy G, Cokugras FC, et al. Lactoferrin levels in the gastric tissue of Helicobacter pylori-positive and -negative patients and its effect on anemia. Mediators Inflamm. 2012;2012:214581. PubMed PMID: 22529520. Pubmed Central PMCID: Pmc3316978. Epub 2012/04/25. eng.

[84] Gold BD, Gilger MA, Czinn SJ. New Diagnostic Strategies for Detection of Helicobacter pylori Infection in Pediatric Patients. Gastroenterol Hepatol (N Y). 2014 Dec; 10(12 Suppl 7):1-19. PubMed PMID: 26491414. Pubmed Central PMCID: Pmc4606978. Epub 2015/10/23. eng.

[85] Mazzucco KL, Junior LM, Lemos NE, Wieck A, Pezzi A, Laureano AM, et al. Assessment of regulatory T cells in childhood immune thrombocytopenic purpura. ISRN Hematol. 2013;2013:143687. PubMed PMID: 24298390. Pubmed Central PMCID: Pmc3835721. Epub 2013/12/04. eng.

[86] Celkan T. Changes in childhood ITP treatment and follow-up in 2011. 2012.

[87] Wilson D. Acquired platelets defects. In: Sciences EH, editor. Nathan and Oski's Hematology of Infancy and Childhood 7th edition. 12009. p. 1553-90.

[88] Evim MS, Baytan B, Gunes AM. Childhood Immune Thrombocytopenia: Long-term Follow-up Data Evaluated by the Criteria of the International Working Group on Immune Thrombocytopenic Purpura. Turk J Haematol. 2014 Mar;31(1):32-9. PubMed PMID: 24764727. Pubmed Central PMCID: Pmc3996642. Epub 2014/04/26. eng.

[89] Provan D, Stasi R, Newland AC, Blanchette VS, Bolton-Maggs P, Bussel JB, et al. International consensus report on the investigation and management of primary immune thrombocytopenia. Blood. 2010 Jan 14;115(2):168-86. PubMed PMID: 19846889. Epub 2009/10/23. eng.

[90] Kuwana M. Helicobacter pylori-associated immune thrombocytopenia: clinical features and pathogenic mechanisms. World J Gastroenterol. 2014 Jan 21;20(3):714-23.

PubMed PMID: 24574745. Pubmed Central PMCID: Pmc3921481. Epub 2014/02/28. eng.

[91] Nugent DJ. Immune thrombocytopenic purpura of childhood. Hematology Am Soc Hematol Educ Program. 2006:97-103. PubMed PMID: 17124046. Epub 2006/11/25. eng.

[92] Nishimoto T, Kuwana M. CD4+CD25+Foxp3+ regulatory T cells in the pathophysiology of immune thrombocytopenia. Semin Hematol. 2013 Jan;50 Suppl 1:S43-9. PubMed PMID: 23664516. Epub 2013/05/17. eng.

[93] McMillan R, Wang L, Tomer A, Nichol J, Pistillo J. Suppression of in vitro megakaryocyte production by antiplatelet autoantibodies from adult patients with chronic ITP. Blood. 2004 Feb 15;103(4):1364-9. PubMed PMID: 14576051. Epub 2003/10/25. eng.

[94] Chang M, Nakagawa PA, Williams SA, Schwartz MR, Imfeld KL, Buzby JS, et al. Immune thrombocytopenic purpura (ITP) plasma and purified ITP monoclonal autoantibodies inhibit megakaryocytopoiesis in vitro. Blood. 2003 Aug 1;102(3):887-95. PubMed PMID: 12676790. Epub 2003/04/05. eng.

[95] Cooper N, Bussel J. The pathogenesis of immune thrombocytopaenic purpura. Br J Haematol. 2006 May;133(4):364-74. PubMed PMID: 16643442. Epub 2006/04/29. eng.

[96] Byrne MF, Kerrigan SW, Corcoran PA, Atherton JC, Murray FE, Fitzgerald DJ, et al. Helicobacter pylori binds von Willebrand factor and interacts with GPIb to induce platelet aggregation. Gastroenterology. 2003 Jun;124(7):1846-54. PubMed PMID: 12806618. Epub 2003/06/14. eng.

[97] Cines DB, Liebman H, Stasi R. Pathobiology of secondary immune thrombocytopenia. Semin Hematol. 2009 Jan;46(1 Suppl 2):S2-14. PubMed PMID: 19245930. Pubmed Central PMCID: Pmc2682438. Epub 2009/03/31. eng.

[98] Franchini M, Cruciani M, Mengoli C, Pizzolo G, Veneri D. Effect of Helicobacter pylori eradication on platelet count in idiopathic thrombocytopenic purpura: a systematic review and meta-analysis. J Antimicrob Chemother. 2007 Aug;60(2):237-46. PubMed PMID: 17561502. Epub 2007/06/15. eng.

[99] Asahi A, Kuwana M, Suzuki H, Hibi T, Kawakami Y, Ikeda Y. Effects of a Helicobacter pylori eradication regimen on anti-platelet autoantibody response in infected and uninfected patients with idiopathic thrombocytopenic purpura. Haematologica. 2006 Oct;91(10):1436-7. PubMed PMID: 16963398. Epub 2006/09/12. eng.

[100] Rajantie J, Klemola T. Helicobacter pylori and idiopathic thrombocytopenic purpura in children. Blood. 2003 Feb 15;101(4):1660. PubMed PMID: 12560248. Epub 2003/02/01. eng.

[101] Stasi R, Provan D. Helicobacter pylori and Chronic ITP. Hematology Am Soc Hematol Educ Program. 2008:206-11. PubMed PMID: 19074084. Epub 2008/12/17. eng.

[102] Yamanishi S, Iizumi T, Watanabe E, Shimizu M, Kamiya S, Nagata K, et al. Implications for induction of autoimmunity via activation of B-1 cells by Helicobacter pylori urease. Infect Immun. 2006 Jan;74(1):248-56. PubMed PMID: 16368978. Pubmed Central PMCID: Pmc1346662. Epub 2005/12/22. eng.

[103] Yeh JJ, Tsai S, Wu DC, Wu JY, Liu TC, Chen A. P-selectin-dependent platelet aggregation and apoptosis may explain the decrease in platelet count during Helicobacter pylori infection. Blood. 2010 May 27;115(21):4247-53. PubMed PMID: 20097880. Epub 2010/01/26. eng.

[104] Andersson P-O, Wadenvik H. Chronic idiopathic thrombocytopenic purpura (ITP): molecular mechanisms and implications for therapy. Expert Reviews in Molecular Medicine. 2004;6(24):1-17.

[105] Troppan K, Wenzl K, Neumeister P, Deutsch A. Molecular Pathogenesis of MALT Lymphoma. Gastroenterol Res Pract. 2015;2015:102656. PubMed PMID: 25922601. Pubmed Central PMCID: Pmc4397421. Epub 2015/04/30. eng.

[106] Cohen SM, Petryk M, Varma M, Kozuch PS, Ames ED, Grossbard ML. Non-Hodgkin's lymphoma of mucosa-associated lymphoid tissue. Oncologist. 2006 Nov-Dec; 11(10):1100-17. PubMed PMID: 17110630. Epub 2006/11/18. eng.

[107] Claviez A, Meyer U, Dominick C, Beck JF, Rister M, Tiemann M. MALT lymphoma in children: a report from the NHL-BFM Study Group. Pediatr Blood Cancer. 2006 Aug;47(2):210-4. PubMed PMID: 16123999. Epub 2005/08/27. eng.

[108] Hasosah M, Baothman A, Satti M, Kutbi S, Alghamdi K, Jacobson K. Mucosa-associated lymphoid tissue lymphoma of the lacrimal gland: sustained remission after eradication of helicobacter pylori infection. Case Rep Gastrointest Med. 2011;2011:945752. PubMed PMID: 22606434. Pubmed Central PMCID: Pmc3350112. Epub 2011/01/01. eng.

[109] Cesta MF. Normal structure, function, and histology of mucosa-associated lymphoid tissue. Toxicol Pathol. 2006;34(5):599-608. PubMed PMID: 17067945. Epub 2006/10/28. eng.

[110] Gisbert JP, Calvet X. Review article: common misconceptions in the management of Helicobacter pylori-associated gastric MALT-lymphoma. Aliment Pharmacol Ther. 2011 Nov;34(9):1047-62. PubMed PMID: 21919927. Epub 2011/09/17. eng.

[111] Wotherspoon AC, Doglioni C, Diss TC, Pan L, Moschini A, de Boni M, et al. Regression of primary low-grade B-cell gastric lymphoma of mucosa-associated lymphoid tissue type after eradication of Helicobacter pylori. Lancet. 1993 Sep 4;342(8871): 575-7. PubMed PMID: 8102719. Epub 1993/09/04. eng.

[112] Wu TC, Chen LK, Lai CR. Primary gastric lymphoma associated with Helicobacter pylori in a child. J Pediatr Gastroenterol Nutr. 2001 May;32(5):608-10. PubMed PMID: 11429527. Epub 2001/06/29. eng.

[113] Liu H, Ye H, Dogan A, Ranaldi R, Hamoudi RA, Bearzi I, et al. T(11;18)(q21;q21) is associated with advanced mucosa-associated lymphoid tissue lymphoma that expresses nuclear BCL10. Blood. 2001 Aug 15;98(4):1182-7. PubMed PMID: 11493468. Epub 2001/08/09. eng.

[114] Zucca E, Roggero E, Pileri S. B-cell lymphoma of MALT type: a review with special emphasis on diagnostic and management problems of low-grade gastric tumours. Br J Haematol. 1998 Jan;100(1):3-14. PubMed PMID: 9450784. Epub 1998/02/05. eng.

[115] Zucca E, Bertoni F, Roggero E, Cavalli F. The gastric marginal zone B-cell lymphoma of MALT type. Blood. 2000 Jul 15;96(2):410-9. PubMed PMID: 10887100. Epub 2000/07/11. eng.

[116] Ricci C, Holton J, Vaira D. Diagnosis of Helicobacter pylori: invasive and non-invasive tests. Best Pract Res Clin Gastroenterol. 2007;21(2):299-313. PubMed PMID: 17382278. Epub 2007/03/27. eng.

[117] Megraud F, Lehours P. Helicobacter pylori detection and antimicrobial susceptibility testing. Clin Microbiol Rev. 2007 Apr;20(2):280-322. PubMed PMID: 17428887. Pubmed Central PMCID: Pmc1865594. Epub 2007/04/13. eng.

[118] van IMC, Laheij RJ, de Boer WA, Jansen JB. The importance of corpus biopsies for the determination of Helicobacter pylori infection. Neth J Med. 2005 Apr;63(4):141-5. PubMed PMID: 15869042. Epub 2005/05/05. eng.

[119] Garza-Gonzalez E, Perez-Perez GI, Maldonado-Garza HJ, Bosques-Padilla FJ. A review of Helicobacter pylori diagnosis, treatment, and methods to detect eradication. World J Gastroenterol. 2014 Feb 14;20(6):1438-49. PubMed PMID: 24587620. Pubmed Central PMCID: Pmc3925853. Epub 2014/03/04. eng.

[120] Uotani T, Graham DY. Diagnosis of Helicobacter pylori using the rapid urease test. Ann Transl Med. 2015 Jan;3(1):9. PubMed PMID: 25705641. Pubmed Central PMCID: Pmc4293486. Epub 2015/02/24. eng.

[121] Koumi A, Filippidis T, Leontara V, Makri L, Panos MZ. Detection of Helicobacter pylori: A faster urease test can save resources. World J Gastroenterol. 2011 Jan 21;17(3): 349-53. PubMed PMID: 21253394. Pubmed Central PMCID: Pmc3022295. Epub 2011/01/22. eng.

[122] Siavoshi F, Saniee P, Khalili-Samani S, Hosseini F, Malakutikhah F, Mamivand M, et al. Evaluation of methods for H. pylori detection in PPI consumption using culture, rapid urease test and smear examination. Ann Transl Med. 2015 Jan;3(1):11. PubMed PMID: 25705643. Pubmed Central PMCID: Pmc4293475. Epub 2015/02/24. eng.

[123] Chisholm SA, Owen RJ, Teare EL, Saverymuttu S. PCR-based diagnosis of Helicobacter pylori infection and real-time determination of clarithromycin resistance directly from human gastric biopsy samples. J Clin Microbiol. 2001 Apr;39(4):1217-20. PubMed PMID: 11283030. Pubmed Central PMCID: Pmc87913. Epub 2001/04/03. eng.

[124] Savarino V, Vigneri S, Celle G. The 13C urea breath test in the diagnosis of Helicobacter pylori infection. Gut. 1999 Jul;45 Suppl 1:I18-22. PubMed PMID: 10457031. Pubmed Central PMCID: Pmc1766662. Epub 1999/08/24. eng.

[125] Tiryaki Z, Yilmaz-Ciftdogan D, Kasirga E. Diagnostic value of stool antigen and antibody tests for Helicobacter pylori infection in Turkish children with upper gastrointestinal complaints before and after eradication. Turk J Pediatr. 2010 Sep-Oct;52(5): 505-11. PubMed PMID: 21434536. Epub 2011/03/26. eng.

[126] Nguyen TV, Bengtsson C, Nguyen GK, Granstrom M. Evaluation of a novel monoclonal-based antigen-in-stool enzyme immunoassay (Premier Platinum HpSA PLUS) for diagnosis of Helicobacter pylori infection in Vietnamese children. Helicobacter. 2008 Aug;13(4):269-73. PubMed PMID: 18665935. Epub 2008/07/31. eng.

[127] Koletzko S, Richy F, Bontems P, Crone J, Kalach N, Monteiro ML, et al. Prospective multicentre study on antibiotic resistance of Helicobacter pylori strains obtained from children living in Europe. Gut. 2006 Dec;55(12):1711-6. PubMed PMID: 16603633. Pubmed Central PMCID: Pmc1856474. Epub 2006/04/11. eng.

[128] Megraud F. H pylori antibiotic resistance: prevalence, importance, and advances in testing. Gut. 2004 Sep;53(9):1374-84. PubMed PMID: 15306603. Pubmed Central PMCID: Pmc1774187. Epub 2004/08/13. eng.

[129] Siu AL. Screening for Iron Deficiency Anemia in Young Children: USPSTF Recommendation Statement. Pediatrics. 2015 Oct;136(4):746-52. PubMed PMID: 26347426. Epub 2015/09/09. eng.

[130] WHO. Iron deficiency anaemia: assessment, prevention and control - A guide for programme managers 2001. Available from: http://www.who.int/iris/bitstream/10665/66914/http://apps.who.int//iris/bitstream/10665/66914/1/WHO_NHD_01.3.pdf?ua=1.

[131] Recommendations to prevent and control iron deficiency in the United States. Centers for Disease Control and Prevention. MMWR Recomm Rep. 1998 Apr 3;47(Rr-3): 1-29. PubMed PMID: 9563847. Epub 1998/05/01. eng.

[132] Liu X, Wang H, Lv Z, Wang Y, Wang B, Xie Y, et al. Rescue Therapy with a Proton Pump Inhibitor Plus Amoxicillin and Rifabutin for Helicobacter pylori Infection: A Systematic Review and Meta-Analysis. Gastroenterol Res Pract. 2015;2015:415648. PubMed PMID: 26106411. Pubmed Central PMCID: PMC4461753. Epub 2015/06/25. eng.

[133] Basu PP, Rayapudi K, Pacana T, Shah NJ, Krishnaswamy N, Flynn M. A randomized study comparing levofloxacin, omeprazole, nitazoxanide, and doxycycline versus triple therapy for the eradication of Helicobacter pylori. Am J Gastroenterol. 2011 Nov; 106(11):1970-5. PubMed PMID: 21989146. Pubmed Central PMCID: PMC3209586. Epub 2011/10/13. eng.

Chapter 5

# Extraintestinal Manifestations in *Helicobacter pylori* Infection – Iron Deficiency Anemia and *Helicobacter pylori*

Sebahat Basyigit, Ferdane Sapmaz, Metin Uzman and Ayse Kefeli

Additional information is available at the end of the chapter

http://dx.doi.org/10.5772/62256

**Abstract**

Iron is an essential element for all living organisms. Iron metabolism is mainly controlled by its absorption. Iron deficiency (ID) is the most common nutritional deficiency, causing important clinical outcomes. One of the most common results of ID is iron deficiency anemia (IDA). The ID results from increased physiological needs, blood losses, inadequate intake, and diminished absorption. *Helicobacter pylori (H. pylori)* infection is one of the important causes of IDA, especially in undetermined and refractory cases.

In the literature, case series, sero-epidemiological studies, and meta-analyses showed robust evidence about the relationship between IDA and *H. pylori*. Several mechanisms have been proposed for IDA in *H. pylori* infection. In this chapter, we review clinical evidence regarding the relationships between *H. pylori* and IDA, iron metabolism, possible mechanisms of IDA in *H. pylori* infection, factors involved in IDA development in *H. pylori* infection, and IDA management in *H. pylori* infection.

**Keywords:** *Helicobacter pylori*,, iron deficiency anemia, hepcidin

## 1. Introduction

Iron (Fe) is an essential element for hemoglobin synthesis, oxidation–reduction reactions, and cellular proliferation. The term iron deficiency (ID) describes a deficit in total body iron, resulting in reduction of serum ferritin levels below normal limit [1]. ID is the most frequent nutritional deficiency worldwide.

ID is associated with impaired cognitive function, diminished work productivity, and behavioral problems in adults and children. In pregnant women, ID has been linked with increased risk for low birth weight, prematurity, and maternal morbidity [2].

Iron deficiency anemia (IDA) is defined as low hemoglobin and plasma ferritin values caused by further decrease in iron stores. IDA is the most common form of anemia worldwide with a prevalence varying from 2% to 8% in developed countries. IDA may occur at all stages of the life cycle, but it is more prevalent in mothers and young children [3].

The known causes of ID are inadequate dietary intake, increased physiological needs as seen in pregnancy and children during rapid growth, increased losses such as bleeding or hemolysis, and diminished iron absorption as seen in celiac disease and chronic inflammatory diseases [4, 5]. Because IDA can result from both physiological and pathological events, the etiology underlying IDA should be determined. The exact cause could not be identified in 20% of cases, despite all routine examinations including gastrointestinal endoscopy and serologic markers for celiac disease [3].

*Helicobacter pylori* (*H. pylori*) infection has been proven as a cause of IDA, especially in undetermined cases. Exact mechanism for IDA in *H. pylori* infection is still unclear. However, several mechanisms have been proposed to explain the relationship between *H. pylori* infection and IDA, including gastrointestinal bleeding and bacterial competition for dietary iron and subversion of the human iron regulatory mechanism [6]. In this chapter, we review clinical evidence regarding the relationship between *H. pylori* and IDA, iron metabolism, possible mechanisms of IDA in *H. pylori* infection, factors involved in the development of IDA in *H. pylori* infection, and IDA management in *H. pylori* infection

## 2. Clinical evidences on the relationship between iron deficiency anemia and *H. pylori*

The relationship between *H. pylori* and IDA was first described by Blecker et al. in 1991. Authors described a 15-year-old patient with IDA due to *H. pylori*-positive chronic active hemorrhagic gastritis without prior gastrointestinal manifestations. Hemoglobin value and serum ferritin level of the patient returned to normal limits unless administration of supplementary iron, after the infection was eradicated [7]. Subsequently, Bruel et al. in 1993 reported a second IDA case (hemoglobin 5.6 g/dL) in an 11-year-old child with *H. pylori* infection complicated with severe digestive hemorrhage. The anemia resolved after the eradication of the *H. pylori* infection without iron replacement [8]. In the same year, the first case with refractory IDA without the symptomatic gastrointestinal pathology was reported in a 7-year-old child by Dufour et al., in which *H. pylori* infection was diagnosed. After the infection was eradicated without supplementary iron treatment, improvement in hematological parameters was observed on month six [9].

Following above-mentioned reports [7-9], further isolated case reports were published in both adolescents and adults in the literature during the 1990s, indicating an association between IDA and *H. pylori* with therapeutic response after *H. pylori* eradication [10-13].

These preliminary case series in the literature encouraged the epidemiologic studies regarding the association between *H. pylori* and IDA. While some studies showed an association between *H. pylori and IDA* among women [14], the other studies showed differences in serum iron levels among *H. pylori*-infected men [15]. In another large cross-sectional study, it was found that *H. pylori* infection was associated with reduction in serum ferritin levels and that this association seemed stronger among adolescents and women at childbearing age [16]. Most epidemiologic studies had cross-sectional design. However, national health surveys enhanced the results of previous reports. Among these, a German study [17] on adult population found a decrease in serum ferritin levels by 16% in individuals infected with *H. pylori* [17]. In addition, children and adolescents were also studied in population-based surveys in South Korea [18-20]. Likewise, these studies showed an association between *H. pylori* and ID. A recent German study on pregnant women reported an association between current *H. pylori* infection and hemoglobin levels [21].

In this category, the largest study was conducted on 7,462 participants aged >3 years from the 1999–2000 National Health and Nutrition Examination Survey (NHANES). The study showed that *H. pylori* infection diagnosed by serology is associated with an increase by 40% in the prevalence of ID in the United States [22].

Finally, meta-analyses have supported the association between *H. pylori* infection and IDA [23-27]. Furthermore, resolution of iron deficiency anemia has been shown following the successful eradication of *H. pylori* [26].

All these publications have supported the relationship between *H. pylori* and IDA.

## 3. Regulation of iron balance

Steps in iron metabolism and contributing molecules are important for understanding effect of *H. pylori* infection on IDA.

Body iron metabolism is a semi-closed system and is critically regulated by several factors. The total amount of body iron is approximately 3–4 g. Two thirds of iron is found in the pool of red blood cell (RBC) and recycled by RBC destruction; the remainder is stored. Only 1–2 mg of iron is absorbed from intestinal tract and circulated in the blood. Since, there is no active mechanism to excrete iron from the body, iron balance is controlled by absorption [1].

Nearly all absorption of dietary iron occurs in the duodenum. Steps involved in iron metabolism include the reduction of iron into a ferrous state ($Fe^{2+}$), apical uptake, intracellular storage or transcellular trafficking, and basolateral release. Several proteins play a role in these steps [Table 1].

| Function | Protein |
|---|---|
| Enzyme | Ferri-reductase |
| | Hemeoxygenase-1 (HO-1) |
| Transport | Divalent metal transporter-1 (DMT-1) |
| | Lipocalin-2 |
| | Ferroportin-1 |
| | Heme-carrier protein-1 |
| | Transferrin |
| | Transferrin receptor 1 / 2 |
| | Natural resistance associated macrophage protein-1 |
| | Hephaestin |
| Storage | Hemosiderin |
| | Ferritin |
| | Lactoferrin |
| Regulatory | Iron regulatory protein 1/2 (IRP) |
| | Iron regulatory elements (IRE) |
| | Hepcidin |

**Table 1.** Proteins Involved in Iron Metabolism

Dietary iron is found in two forms; heme iron (10%) that is derived from meat and bound to hemoglobin (Hb) and myoglobin and nonheme iron (90%) that is ionic and inorganic in form derived from plants (Figure 1). Both iron forms are absorbed at the apical surface of duodenal cells through different mechanisms.

Nonheme iron taken on a diet presents initially in oxidized (ferric-$Fe^{3+}$) form. This form of iron is not bioavailable, and before it is absorbed by an enterocyte it needs to be reduced to the $Fe^{2+}$ form via ferri-reductase enzyme [28]. $Fe^{3+}$ reduction is optimized by low gastric pH. Gastric acid, dietary ascorbic acid, and luminal reductases enhance the iron absorption [29]. Iron is transported across the intestinal epithelium by a transporter called divalent metal transporter-1 (DMT-1) that also transports other metal ions by a proton-coupled mechanism [30] (Figure 1). There is also a siderophore-like iron uptake pathway mediated by lipocalin-2 that seems to exert an innate immune response against bacterial infection by sequestrating iron. However, physiological role of lipocalin-2 has not been fully elucidated.

Heme iron is better absorbed than nonheme form. Heme iron is absorbed into enterocytes by heme carrier protein-1 that is a membrane protein found in the proximal intestine [31] (Figure 1). Heme iron is degraded by hemeoxygenase-1 (HO-1) within enterocyte [32] (Figure 1).

In the intestinal epithelial cell, iron can follow two pathways. Firstly, it may remain in the cell to be used or stored. This iron is excreted when intestinal cells demise and are molted into the lumen. Secondly, iron is transported into circulation from basolateral membrane of the enterocyte. This part is called absorbed iron. Ferroportin-1 is the sole supposed iron exporter that has been defined so far. $Fe^{2+}$ is transported from the basal membrane via ferroportin-1;

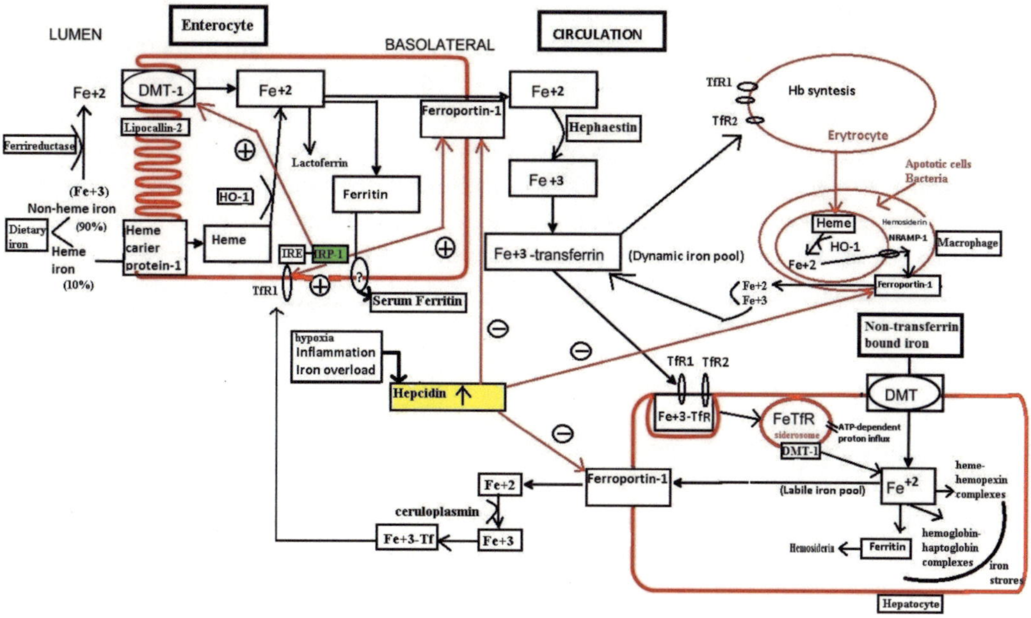


**Figure 1.** Regulation of Iron Balance

thereafter, it is oxidized into $Fe^{3+}$ by a multi-copper-oxidase protein called hephaestin, an enzymatic protein similar to plasma ceruloplasmin, before being bound by plasma transferrin (Tf). Ferroportin-1 is also the putative iron exporter in macrophages and hepatocytes [1, 28].

Iron absorption, mediated by two models, is up-regulated by iron deficiency and increased erythropoiesis or down-regulated in inflammation and iron repletion. These two models can be entitled as crypt programming model and the hepcidin model.

**The crypt programming model:** The intracellular iron level of the duodenal crypt cells intercommunicate with the iron deposits of the body, which, in turn, establishes the amount of iron absorbed from the intestinal lumen. The crypt cells express both transferrin receptor-1 (TfR1) and TfR2. The cellular uptake of Tf-bound iron from plasma is mediated by these receptors [28, 33].

TfR1 is expressed pervasively and Tf-mediated iron uptake is proposed to take place in majority of the cell types. Despite that, expression of TfR2 is limited in hepatocytes, duodenal crypt cells, and erythroid cells, suggesting a more privatized mission in iron balance.

Iron regulatory elements (IREs) act as iron sensors and regulate translation or stability of mRNA-encoding proteins. The intracellular iron level commands the interaction of IREs with cytosolic iron regulatory proteins (IRPs) 1 and 2. In the absence of iron, IRP1 binds to IREs of TfR1, DMT-1, and ferroportin-1 mRNA; then, syntheses of these proteins begin in the duodenum and dietary iron absorption is increased. Thus, increased IRP-binding activity represents decreased body iron stores [28].

**The hepcidin model:** Liver hepcidin is a 25-amino-acid cysteine-rich peptide. Numerous factors contribute to the regulation of hepcidin level. Liver iron levels, inflammation, hypoxia, and anemia can be counted among these factors. Hepcidin regulates the rate of iron absorption by controlling the expression of ferroportin-1 at basolateral membranes of enterocytes. Internalization of ferroportin-1 and loss of its function occur after the binding of hepcidin to ferroportin-1. Ferroportin-1 molecules take place also in macrophages and liver. Hence, it is suggested that iron release from intestinal crypt cells, liver, and macrophages is reduced, when hepcidin levels are increased in iron overload or inflammation (*via* IL-6). In contrast, it is likely that ferroportin-1 expression and iron release is increased when hepcidin levels are reduced as is the case in ID, anemia or hypoxia [34].

Iron released into the circulation binds to Tf and is transported to sites of use and storage. Three forms of Tf can be found in plasma: apo-transferrin that contains no iron, monoferric-transferrin, and diferric-transferrin. About 30–40% of these iron-binding Tf sites are occupied under normal physiological conditions. Tf-bound iron is the most important dynamic iron pool [35]. Tf-bound iron enters into target cells, mainly erythroid cells, but also immune and hepatic cells via a process of receptor-mediated endocytosis [28]. Tf binds to receptor, which is called TfR and located on the plasma membrane. Siderosomes, clathrin-coated endosomes, are formed by invagination of Tf and receptor–ligand complexes at the cell-surface membrane [35]. After that, the siderosomes are acidified by an ATP-dependent proton influx. This process leads to conformational changes in Tf and TFR1, and promotes iron release of $Fe^{3+}$ from Tf. Then, $Fe^{3+}$ is converted to $Fe^{2+}$ through a ferri-reductase and moved to the cytoplasm by the DMT-1, while the TfR is appraised at the cell membrane again and Tf is drained back to the circulation [28, 36]. Production of hemoglobin by the erythron accounts for most iron use. High-level expression of TfR1 in erythroid precursors ensures the uptake of iron into this compartment.

Hemoglobin iron has an important cycle, as aging erythrocytes undergo phagocytosis. In the phagocytic vesicles of reticuloendothelial system macrophages, heme is metabolized through heme oxygenase-1 (HO-1). Then, iron is released to the cytoplasm by natural-resistance-associated macrophage protein-1, a transport protein similar to DMT-1. Macrophages are also able to gain iron from other apoptotic cells and bacteria [1]. Iron is stored in two forms in the cell: as ferritin in the cytosol and as hemosiderin originated from degradation of ferritin within the lysosomes. Hemosiderin is a very small part of body iron stores. It is found mostly in macrophages and increases in iron overload [35]. Iron export from macrophages to Tf is accomplished primarily by ferroportin-1, the same iron-export protein expressed in duodenal enterocytes, and hephaestin [28] (Figure 1). The amount of iron required for daily production of 300 billion RBCs (20–30 mg) is mostly provided by recycling of iron by macrophages [1].

The liver is a major storage organ of iron, in which excess iron is stored as ferritin and hemosiderin. The uptake of Tf-bound iron by the liver from plasma is mediated by TfR1 and TfR2. In iron overload states, Tf is saturated and redundant iron is found in the form of non-Tf-bound iron. This form of iron is transported along with the hepatocyte membrane through a carrier-mediated process compatible with DMT-1. The hepatocytes can also warehouse iron as ferritin, hemoglobin–haptoglobin complexes, and heme–hemopexin complexes. Whereas, ferroportin-1 is known to be the only protein that mediates the iron transport from hepatocytes. Iron is oxidized by ceruloplasmin and attached to Tf after being released from hepatocytes [1, 28] (Figure 1).

Iron is also found at mucosal surfaces as lactoferrin. In addition to these proteins, an additional fraction of free iron is present in the form of the labile iron pool within cells.

## 4. Possible mechanisms of iron deficiency in *H. pylori* infection

The mechanisms by which *H. pylori* infection contributes to IDA remain unclear. Several studies have suggested different biologic mechanisms by which infection with *H. pylori* may induce depletion in the iron stores of the host. Four explanations can be posted: 1) overt or occult blood loss due to gastroduodenal lesions [37]; 2) decreased iron absorption due to hypo- or achlorhydria [38]; 3) increased iron consumption by *H. pylori* [39]; and 4) iron sequestration into the gastric mucosa [40,Table 2].

| Mechanism | Findings |
|---|---|
| Blood loss | Peptic ulcer diseases<br>Gastric carcinoma<br>Gastric lymphoma<br>Chronic erosive esophagitis,<br>Chronic erosive gastritis<br>Chronic erosive duodenitis |
| Malabsorption of iron | Atrophic gastritis<br>Reversible hypoclorhydria |
| Bacterial competition for iron | |
| Changing molecular mechanisms in iron metabolism | Elevated hepcidin level<br>Decreased hemeoxygenase-1<br>Mislocalization of transferrin receptor |

**Table 2.** Possible Mechanisms of Iron Deficiency in *Helicobacter pylori* Infection

### 4.1. Blood loss from gastrointestinal lesions

Blood loss is the most important cause of iron deficiency in adults. Each milliliter of blood loss (if Hb is 15 g/dL) results in loss of 0.5 mg of iron approximately. Gastrointestinal blood loss is the most important cause in postmenopausal women and men. While menstrual blood loss commonly causes IDA in premenopausal women, coexistent gastrointestinal lesions have often been identified [3].

IDA resulting from gastrointestinal bleeding is a common feature of many gastrointestinal conditions. The most common cause of upper gastrointestinal bleeding is peptic ulcer bleeding, which is responsible for about 50% of all cases, followed by esophagitis and erosive disease [41].

*H. pylori* infection is associated with both duodenal and gastric ulcer disease. Subjects infected with *H. pylori* have an average lifetime risk of 10–20% for the occurrence of peptic ulcer disease. This risk is at least three- to fourfold higher than in noninfected individuals. The bacteria can be determined in 90–100% of subjects with duodenal ulcer and in 60–100% of subjects with gastric ulcer. Individuals infected with bacterial strain producing a cytotoxin, or owning cytotoxin-associated gene A (cagA), have a higher risk of development of peptic ulcer disease. Other factors affecting the risk of peptic ulcer disease in infected individuals are amount of gastric acid production, gastric metaplasia in the duodenal bulb, smoking, and genetic factors (e.g., blood group O and lack of the secretor gene) [42]. Testing for *H. pylori* is recommended in all patients with peptic ulcer bleeding [43]; eradication therapy for those who are *H. pylori*-positive and then evaluation of the effect of this therapy. Retreatment with subsequent regimen should also be considered in the patients who had eradication failure. The effectiveness of eradication treatment and maintenance antisecretory therapy for the prevention of rebleeding has been evaluated in several studies. A meta-analysis showed that *H. pylori* eradication group had significantly decreased risk of rebleeding; even when only patients with successful *H. pylori* eradication were evaluated, the rebleeding rate was found significantly lower [44]. Thus, confirmation of eradication should be tested. Diagnostic tests for *H. pylori* have a low negative predictive value in case of active bleeding [45]. Thus, initial negative results on biopsies obtained in the acute setting should be judged with caution and repetition of the test during follow-up is recommended [43].

Gastric carcinoma is also one of the important causes of gastrointestinal bleeding accounting for nearly 4–8% of all cases [46]. The most common histopathological features of gastric malignancies are adenocarcinoma and lymphoma of mucosa- associated lymphoid tissue (MALT). Approximately 90% of gastric tumors are adenocarcinoma, whereas gastric MALT lymphomas are considerably less common (approximately 3% of all gastric tumors) [47]. *H. pylori* infection plays an important carcinogenic role in both gastric carcinoma and MALT lymphoma [48]. It has been calculated that the risk for gastric adenocarcinoma and MALT lymphoma is three- to sixfold higher in *H. pylori*-infected individuals than those who are noninfected [47]. Because of the strong association between gastric cancer and *H. pylori* infection, the World Health Organization (WHO) classified *H. pylori* as a class I carcinogen in 1994 [49]. In gastric carcinogenesis, host-related genetic elements such as a pro-inflammatory cytokine profile and/or a positive family history as well as bacterial virulence factors play important roles. Furthermore, environmental factors, like nutrition, and socioeconomic factors are suggested to be also important. After the initiation by *H. pylori* and the influence of variable environmental and host factors, chronic active gastritis may progressively evolve to atrophic gastritis and intestinal metaplasia. In some individuals, the metaplastic epithelium will undergo further genomic and phenotypic changes, resulting in gastric dysplasia and eventual adenocarcinoma [50]. The "test and treat" strategy for *H. pylori* infection should be considered effective for prevention of gastric carcinoma only in communities with a high incidence of gastric carcinoma [51].

*H. pylori* has been identified as causative agent for chronic erosive gastritis, erosive esophagitis, and erosive duodenitis [52-54]. These lesions are also among the important causes of occult gastrointestinal bleeding [3].

### 4.2. Decreased iron absorption secondary to hypo- or achlorhydria

Iron malabsorption is one of the most important causes of IDA. Decreased iron absorption may result from intestinal mucosal disorders (most frequently, celiac disease), impaired gastric acid secretion (including use of proton pump inhibitors), and gastric/intestinal bypass procedures [3].

As mentioned above, nonheme ferric iron is required to be reduced to a ferrous form before its absorption in the duodenum and first jejunum. Gastric acid has an important role in reducing and solubilizing the inorganic form of the iron [30]. Ferric iron has been demonstrated to be insoluble and precipitates at pH above 3 [55]. Thus, IDA can develop in patients with hypochlorhydria because of gastric surgery or atrophic body gastritis [56, 57].

Atrophic body gastritis is characterized by atrophy of the gastric body mucosa, hypergastrinemia, and hypo-achlorhydria [58]. Atrophy is a time-related phenomenon and *H. pylori* infection is considered an etiologic factor in the development of atrophic body gastritis [59]. This can eventually lead to loss of gastric glands and development of multifocal atrophic gastritis, which is often accompanied by intestinal metaplasia. A steady increase in the prevalence of atrophy and metaplasia is seen with advancing age [60]. As with peptic ulcer disease, the chance for development of atrophic body gastritis depends on the severity of gastritis and the characteristics of the bacterial strain [59]. Another interesting factor that can influence the development of atrophic body gastritis is *H. pylori* lipopolysaccharide mimicking Lewis x and y antigens. The presence of cross-reacting antibodies against the antigens and the gastric mucosa may have a great chance to develop atrophy [61]. Atrophic body gastritis may improve on long-term follow-up after *H. pylori* eradication, which is thus strongly recommended in atrophic gastritis [62].

It is well known that *H. pylori* infection induces gastric acid hyposecretion irrespective of presence of fundus atrophy when affecting the gastric body [63]. Also, *H. pylori* gastritis has been demonstrated to be associated with a reversible reduction in the ascorbic acid levels of gastric juice [64]. Therefore, a diffuse *H. pylori*-gastritis could decrease iron absorption by altering the physiological gastric secretion, even if it is mild [65].

### 4.3. Increased iron uptake and utilization by bacteria

*H. pylori* has been shown as a causative agent in IDA that is not attributable to usual reasons such as intestinal losses or poor intake, malabsorption or diversion of iron in the reticuloendothelial system, and unresponsive to iron therapy. The possible mechanism may be explained via bacterial competition for dietary iron.

Iron is an essential trace element in all organisms, even for pathogenic bacteria. Acquisition of iron by *H. pylori* from the host is necessary for colonization and infection [66]. Intracellular bacterial iron is exactly regulated and kept at an optimal level. Mostly, the free iron in the host is found to be complexes with proteins such as Tf and lactoferrin on mucosal surfaces. Thus, the available extracellular host iron is at a very low level. Therefore, bacterial pathogens such as *H. pylori* have to develop some mechanisms to compete for the restricted extracellular iron in the host to survive and maintain disease [67, 68].

In the gastric mucosa, iron is available as lactoferrin, heme compounds arising from damaged tissues, and iron based on pepsin-degraded food. Iron represents increased solubility in the acidic fluid, and iron-complexing proteins of eukaryotic organisms exhibit lower binding capacity under the acidic conditions in gastric juice.

*H. pylori* produce several iron transport proteins and iron storage proteins [69-72,Table 3]. $Fe^{2+}$ is the main form of free iron in the gastric medium, and *H. pylori* keeps this ferrous ion through the FeoB protein [73]. FeoB-mediated iron acquisition has great importance for *H. pylori*. It has been shown that isogenic FeoB mutant mice could not colonize the gastric mucosa [73]. Ferric reductase activity for conversion of $Fe^{3+}$ to $Fe^{2+}$ is transported by the FeoB system of *H. pylori* [74].

| Function | Protein |
|---|---|
| Enzyme | Ferri-reductase |
| | Hemeoxygenase-1 (HugZ) |
| Transport | FeoB |
| | FecA (ferric citrate outer membrane receptor) |
| | FecD (inner membrane permease) |
| | FecE (ATP-binding protein) |
| | FrpB (outer membrane receptor) |
| | CeuE (periplasmic-binding protein) |
| | Iron repressible outer membrane proteins (IROMPs) |
| | Lactoferrin-binding protein |
| | Siderophore |
| Storage | Pfr-ferritin |
| | *Helicobacter pylori*-neutrophil-activating protein-(HP-NAP)- |
| | Bacterioferritin |

**Table 3.** Proteins Involved in Iron Acquision System of *Helicobacter pylori*

Additionally, *H. pylori* also has various transport systems for ferric iron [72, 75]. Since the ferric iron is insoluble, its transport needs an outer membrane receptor to transport the iron over the outer membrane. *H. pylori* has three copies of the ferric citrate outer membrane receptor FecA and three copies of the FrpB outer membrane receptor [69-72]. There are two copies of the periplasmic-binding protein CeuE and finally a single inner membrane permease (FecD) and an ATP-binding protein (FecE). ABC transporter system transports the iron from the periplasm to the cytoplasm [73].

Subsequently, specific outer membrane receptor proteins bind the iron. It has been suggested that heme-iron-repressible outer membrane proteins (IROMPs) are involved in heme binding and/or uptake by *H. pylori* [39]. When the heme is located in the cytoplasm, it can be used by a heme oxygenase protein. Heme oxygenase catalyzes the NADPH-reductase-dependent degradation of heme to biliverdin, which is the rate-limiting step leading to the release of iron and carbon monoxide. Some researchers have identified a heme oxygenase protein called HugZ that is responsible for heme iron utilization in *H. pylori* [76].

A common iron acquisition system present in many pathogens is the secretion of low-molecular-mass, high-affinity iron chelators, which are called siderophores. These chelators are able to remove iron from Tf or lactoferrin [77-78].

Two iron storage proteins in *H. pylori* have been characterized, the Pfr ferritin and *H. pylori* neutrophil-activating protein (HP-NAP) bacterioferritin. The 19-kDa Pfr ferritin serves as an intracellular iron deposit and protects *H. pylori* against iron toxicity and free iron-mediated oxidative stress [79-83]. Iron-binding Pfr ferritin can be delivered and reused to maintain growing up in the iron-limited states [83]. HP-NAP was isolated from neutrophilic granulocytes as an immuno-dominant protein in vitro [84]. It was demonstrated to mediate adhesion of *H. pylori* to mucin [85]. The HP-NAP protein is similar to bacterioferritins [86, 87]. Although it is suggested, a role of HP-NAP in *H. pylori* iron storage is yet to be demonstrated [87].

In addition, lactoferrin-binding protein has been suggested to be highly specific for human lactoferrin in *H. pylori* infection [40].

All these mechanisms suggest that *H. pylori* utilize the iron from host and use or store for colonization and growth.

### 4.4. Changing molecular mechanisms in iron metabolism

*H. pylori* may act in changing molecular mechanisms that play a role in iron metabolism.

The best evaluated molecule in the association between *H. pylori* and ID is hepcidin. Hepcidin is a protein that is secreted into the blood and interacts with villous enterocytes to regulate the rate of iron absorption by controlling the expression of ferroportin-1. When hepcidin is increased, iron release from enterocytes is reduced. The anemia of chronic inflammation is mediated, in part, by the stimulation of hepcidin by cytokines [35]. Hepcidin has been reported to be elevated in patients infected with *H. pylori,* acting as an acute-phase reactant in response to the inflammation produced in the gastric mucosa and resulting in a pathology known as "anemia of inflammation or chronic disease" [88-90]. Prohepcidin, hepcidin's precursor, was also shown to increase in *H. pylori* infection and is decreased after eradication of *H. pylori* infection [91].

HO-1 is an enzyme that is responsible in heme degradation in host enterocytes. *H. pylori* may affect levels of HO-1. A significant increase in Keap1 gene expression was found in transfected AGS cells with *H. pylori* HspB. The increase in Keap1 was associated to decreased antioxidant enzymes including HO-1, and phase II detoxifying enzyme NAD(P)H:quinone oxidoreductase-1 [92]. CagA status is suggested to be important in this action of *H. pylori.* HO-1 is also found to be down-regulated in gastric epithelial cells of patients infected with cagA-positive *H. pylori* but not in gastric epithelial cells of patients infected with cagA-negative *H. pylori* [93].

TfR1 and TfR2 on cell surface mediate the cellular uptake of Tf-bound iron from plasma [28]. *H. pylori* is known to affect host cell polarity and intracellular trafficking [94]. In *H. pylori*-infected cell lines, it has been shown that Tfr was mislocalized to sites of *H. pylori* microcolony growth at the apical cell surface. *H. pylori* colonization of the polarized epithelium has been shown to lead to increased apical release of Tf [95].

## 5. Factors that affect iron deficiency development in *H. pylori* infection

Although *H. pylori* gastric infection has been shown to be strongly associated with IDA, it is only a small portion of patients with *H. pylori* gastritis that develop IDA. The main question is why only a small portion of patients with *H. pylori* gastritis develop IDA, and what differentiates these patients.

The pattern of *H. pylori*-related gastritis is a significant predictor of the results of infection, and it determines the different effects of the bacteria on gastric functions. The panelists of the updated Sydney system suggested that most individuals infected with *H. pylori* develop a more evident inflammation in the antrum (nearly double) compared to the corpus in the absence of atrophy [96].

The relationship between chronic gastritis and gastric acid secretion is strictly dependent on the topography of gastric inflammation [97]. It has been demonstrated that gastritis in the corporal mucosa leads to decreased acid secretion with a consequent increase in intragastric pH [98]. Severity of inflammation is also important in terms of clinical outcomes.

Additionally, *H. pylori* strains owning the cagA or the vacuolating cytotoxin A (vacA), which are highly virulent, display potent mechanisms to produce or magnify ID in patients comparing less virulent strains [99, 100]. For example, Baysoy et al. have reported that cagA-positive strains was associated with a greater decrease in gastric juice ascorbic acid compared to cagA-negative strains [101]. Tan et al. reported that cagA and vacA contribute to iron uptake from gastric epithelial cells in a cooperative manner. VacA induces apical mislocalization of TfR. CagA alters internalization and intracellular transport of TfR. These pathogenic factors take away iron from holo-transferrin of host and maintain colonization on the gastric epithelial cell surface [95]. Moreover, Cardenas et al. found that patients infected with the cagA-positive strains did not improve their ferritin levels after eradication treatment as much as those who were cagA-negative [102].

## 6. Management of iron deficiency in *H. pylori* infection

Like other hematological conditions such as MALT lymphoma, vitamin B12 deficiency, and idiopathic thrombocytopenic purpura, IDA is also included in the international consensus and guidelines as an indication for "test and treat" of *H. pylori* [51, 62, 103,Table 4]. Whereas, it should not substitute the other workup for IDA. The endoscopic evaluations for upper and lower gastrointestinal tracts in men and postmenaposal women, celiac serology should be performed in cases of IDA.

| Hematological Condition | Level of Evidence |
|---|---|
| MALT lymphoma | Evidence level: 1a Grade of recommendation: A |
| IDA | Evidence level: 1a<br>Grade of recommendation: A |
| Idiopathic thrombocytopenic purpura | Evidence level: 1b<br>Grade of recommendation: A |
| Vitamin B12 deficiency | Evidence level: 3b<br>Grade of recommendation: B |

Abbrevations: Grades of recommendations and evidence levels in support of recommendations
Grade of recommendation: A; Evidence level: 1a: Systematic review of randomized controlled trial (RCT) of goog methodological quality and with homogeneity
Grade of recommendation: A; Evidence level: 1b: Individual RCT with narrow CI
Grade of recommendation: B; Evidence level: 3b: Individual case-control study

**Table 4.** Evidence Based Relationship between *H. pylori* and the Etiology of other Hematological Conditions (in these disorders, *H. pylori* should be sought and eradicated)

It is possible to rescue hematological and ferro-kinetic parameters after *H. pylori* eradication. Its implication as an unexplained origin of ID was revealed in the international consensus and management guidelines of *H. pylori* infection. It should be tested and eradicated in both adults and children with unexplained origin of ID [104,105].

There has not been any concensus on the treatment of IDA in *H. pylori*-infected patients yet. Three meta-analyses evaluated the effect of *H. pylori* eradication on IDA. Qu et al. reported that eradication of *H. pylori* improved hemoglobin and serum ferritin levels but not significantly [27]. Whereas, Huang et al. reported another meta-analysis of 8 randomized controlled trials (RCTs) in which five RCTs had used PPI-based triple therapy and three RCTs had used bismuth-based triple therapy as eradication regimens. They found that anti-*H. pylori* treatment combined with iron supplement was more effective than iron administration alone in the treatment of IDA in *H. pylori*-infected patients. They also showed that bismuth-based triple therapy had an advantage over PPI-based triple therapy [26]. However, this finding needs to be confirmed. In another meta-analysis involving 956 patients and 16 RCTs in which 13 RCT had used PPI-based triple treatment and 3 RCT used bismuth-based triple treatment, it was shown that the increase in Hb, serum iron, and serum ferritin levels were significantly higher with anti-*H. pylori* treatment plus oral iron compared with oral iron alone in patients with documented *H. pylori* infection and IDA [24]. Recently in a study by Habib et al., sequential and standard therapies were compared in children. It was shown that there was no significant difference in *H. pylori* eradication success between two groups and there was no significant relationship between eradication treatment and serum ferritin levels [106].

In conclusion, refractoriness to oral iron treatment and unexplained IDA may justify a "test-and-treat" approach of *H. pylori* eradication as recommended by the Maastricht IV European Consensus Conference [62], Second Asia–Pacific Consensus Guideline [51], and the III Working Group Consensus Report 2015 [103]. Standard treatment regimens that are recommended in dyspeptic patients by current guidelines combined with iron supplement are effective in IDA in patients with *H. pylori* infection. These eradication regimens are listed in Table 5 based on current guidelines [Table 5,51, 62, 103].

| **First-line therapy** | **Duration** | **Drugs and doses** |
|---|---|---|
| Standard PPI-based triple therapy | 7-14 days | PPI 2x1<br>+ Amoxicillin 1g 2x1<br>+ Clarithromycin 500 mg 2x1<br>or<br>(in the presence of penicillin allergy)<br>PPI 2x1<br>+ Metronidazole 500 mg 2x1<br>+Clarithromycin 500 mg 2x1<br>or<br>(in areas of low clarithromycin resistance)<br>PPI 2x1<br>+ Amoxicillin 1 g 2x1<br>+ Metronidazole 400 mg 2x1 |
| Sequential therapy | First 5 days | PPI 2x1 + Amoxicillin 1 g 2x1 |
| | Followed by 5 days | PPI 2x1<br>+ Metronidazole or tinidazole 500 mg 2x1<br>+ Clarithromycin 500 mg 2x1 |
| Concomitant therapy<br>(non-bismuth quadruple) | 10 days | PPI 2x1<br>+ Amoxicillin 1g 2x1<br>+ Metronidazole or tinidazole 500mg 2x1<br>+ Clarithromycin 500 mg 2x1 |
| **Second-line therapy** | **Duration** | **Drugs and doses** |
| *Bismuth-containing quadruple therapy<br>(when bismuth is available) | 7–14 days | PPI 2x1<br>+ Bismuth salts 4x1 or 2x2<br>+ Tetracycline, 500mg 3x1<br>+ Metronidazole, 500mg 3x1 |
| Levofloxacin-containing triple therapy | 10 days | PPI 2x1<br>+ Amoxicillin 1g 2x1<br>+ Levofloxacin, 500mg 1x1 or 250mg 2x1<br>or<br>(in the presence of penicillin allergy)<br>PPI 2x1<br>+ Clarithromycin 500 mg 2x1<br>+ Levofloxacin, 500mg 1x1 or 250mg 2x1 |
| Rifabutin-based triple therapy: | 7–10 days | PPI 2x1<br>+Rifabutin 150 mg 2x1<br>+Amoxicillin 1 g 2x1 |
| **Third-line therapy** | | |
| After failure of second-line therapy, treatment should be guided by antimicrobial susceptibility testing, whenever possible | | |

*In areas of high clarithromycin resistance, bismuth-containing quadruple therapy is recommended for first-line empirical treatment.
Abbrevations: PPI: Proton pump inhibitor

**Table 5.** Treatment regimens recommended for first- and second-line therapy of *Helicobacter pylori* infection

## 7. Summary

Iron is an essential element for all living organisms. Iron metabolism is controlled mainly by absorption. ID is the most common nutritional deficiency and causes clinically important outcomes. One of the most common results of ID is IDA. ID results from increased physiological needs, blood losses, inadequate intake, and diminished absorption. *H. pylori* infection is one of the important causes of IDA especially in undetermined and refractory cases.

In the literature case series, sero-epidemiological studies and meta-analysis showed strong evidence regarding the relationship between IDA and *H. pylori*. Several mechanisms have been proposed for IDA in *H. pylori* infection. First, blood loss from gastrointestinal lesions related with *H. pylori*; second, malabsorption due to hypo- or achlorhydria resulting from gastric body inflammation and atrophy; third, bacterial competition for dietary iron with several mechanisms; and last, changing regulatory pathways especially hepcidin levels in iron metabolism by the bacteria.

Although *H. pylori* infection is more prevalent, frequency of IDA related with *H. pylori* is low. Influencing factors for developing IDA in *H. pylori* infection include topographic distribution of gastric inflammation, severity of inflammation, virulence factor of the bacteria.

Once IDA is diagnosed in *H. pylori*-infected patient, other most common causes of IDA should be evaluated carefully. Depending on "test and treat" strategy, the *H. pylori* infection should be eradicated based on recommendations by the current guidelines.

## Author details

Sebahat Basyigit[1*], Ferdane Sapmaz[1], Metin Uzman[1] and Ayse Kefeli[2]

*Address all correspondence to: sbuyuktemiz@yahoo.com

1 Department of Gastroenterology, Kecioren Research and Training Hospital, Ankara, Turkey

2 Department of Gastroenterology, Siirt State Hospital, Siirt, Turkey

## References

[1] Andrews NC. Disorders of iron metabolism. *N Engl J Med* 1999; 341: 1986-1995. DOI: 10.1056/NEJM199912233412607

[2] Pasricha SR, Flecknoe-Brown SC, Allen KJ, Gibson PR, McMahon LP, Olynyk JK, Roger SD, Savoia HF, Tampi R, Thomson AR, Wood EM, Robinson KL. Diagnosis

and management of iron deficiency anaemia: a clinical update. *Med J Aust* 2010; 193(9): 525-532.

[3] Goddard AF, James MW, McIntyre AS, Scott BB. Guidelines for the management of iron deficiency anaemia. *Gut* 2011; 2010: 2-8. DOI:10.1136/gut.2010.228874

[4] Oti-Boateng P, Seshadri R, Petrick S, Gibson RA, Simmer K. Iron status and dietary iron intake of 6–24-month-old children in Adelaide. *J Paediatr Child Health* 1998; 34: 250-253. DOI:10.1046/j.1440-1754.1998.00205.x

[5] Peeling P, Dawson B, Goodman C, Landers G, Trinder D. Athletic induced iron deficiency: new insights into the role of inflammation, cytokines and hormones. *Eur J Appl Physiol* 2008; 103: 381-391. DOI 10.1007/s00421-008-0726-6

[6] Barabino A. Helicobacter pylori related iron deficiency anemia: a review. *Helicobacter* 2002; 7(2): 71-75. DOI:10.1046/j.1083-4389.2002.00073.x

[7] Blecker U, Renders F, Lanciers S, Vandenplas Y. Syncopes leading to the diagnosis of a Helicobacter pylori positive chronic active haemorrhagic gastritis. *Eur J Pediatr* 1991; 150: 560-561. DOI: 10.1007/BF02072207

[8] Bruel H, Dabadie A, Pouedras P, Gambert C, Le Gall E, Jezequel C. Helicobacter pylori gastritis manifested by acute anemia. *Ann Pediatr* (Paris) 1993; 40: 364-367.

[9] Dufour C, Brisigotti M, Fabretti G, Luxardo P, Mori PG, Barabino A. Helicobacter pylori gastric infection and sideropenic refractory anemia. *J Pediatr Gastroenterol Nutr* 1993; 17: 225-227.

[10] Marignani M, Angeletti S, Bordi C, Malagnino F, Mancino C, Delle Fave G. Annibale B. Reversal of long-standing iron deficiency anaemia after eradication of Helicobacter pylori infection. *Scand J Gastroenterol* 1997; 32: 617-622:DOI: DOI: 10.3109/00365529709025109

[11] Barabino A, Dufour C, Marino CE, Claudiani F, De Alessan-dri A. Unexplained refractory iron-deficiency anemia associ-ated with Helicobacter pylori gastric infection in children: further clinical evidence. *J Pediatr Gastroenterol Nutr* 1999; 28: 116-119.

[12] Capurso G, Marignani M, Delle Fave G, Annibale B. Iron-deficiency anemia in premenopausal women: why not consider atrophic body gastritis and Helicobacter pylori role? *Am J Gastroenterol* 1999; 94: 3084-3308. DOI: 10.1111/j.1572-0241.1999.03084.x

[13] Carnicer J, Badia R, Argemi J. Helicobacter pylori gastritis and sideropenic refractory anemia. *J Pediatr Gastroenterol Nutr* 1997; 25(4): 441.

[14] Peach HG, Bath NE, Farish SJ. Helicobacter pylori infection: an added stressor on iron status of women in the community. *Med J Aust* 1998; 69: 188-190.

[15] Collett JA, Burt MJ, Frampton CM, Yeo KH, Chapman TM, Buttimore RC, Cook HB, Chapman BA. Seroprevalence of Helicobacter pylori in the adult population of

Christchurch: risk factors and relationship to dyspeptic symptoms and iron studies. *N Z Med J* 1999; 112: 292-295.

[16] Parkinson AJ, Gold BD, Bulkow L, Wainwright RB, Swaminathan B, Khanna B, Petersen KM, Fitzgerald MA. High prevalence of Helicobacter pylori in the Alaska native population and association with low serum ferritin levels in young adults. *Clin Diagnostic Lab Immunol* 2000; 7(6): 885-888. DOI: 10.1128/CDLI.7.6.885-888.2000

[17] Berg G, Bode G, Blettner M, Boeing H, Brenner H. Helicobacter pylori infection and serum ferritin: a population-based study among 1806 adults in Germany. *Am J Gastroenterol* 2001; 96(4): 1014-1018.DOI: 10.1111/j.1572-0241.2001.03686.x

[18] Choe YH, Kim SK, Son BK, Lee DH, Hong YC, Pai, SH. Randomized placebo-controlled trial of Helicobacter pylori eradication for iron Deficiency anemia in preadolescent children and adolescents. *Helicobacter* 1999; 4(2): 135-139. DOI:10.1046/j.1523-5378.1999.98066.x

[19] Seo JK, Ko JS, Choi KD. Serum ferritin and Helicobacter pylori infection in children: A seroepidemiologic study in Korea. J *Gastroenterol Hepatol* 2002; 17(7): 754-757. DOI: 10.1046/j.1440-1746.2002.02797.x

[20] Choi JW. Does Helicobacter pylori infection relate to iron deficiency anaemia in prepubescent children under 12 years of age?*Acta Paediatrica* 2003; 92(8): 970-972. DOI: 10.1111/j.1651-2227.2003.tb00633.x

[21] Weyermann M, Rothenbacher D, Gayer L, Bode G, Adler G, Grab D, Brenner H. Role of Helicobacter pylori infection in iron deficiency during pregnancy. *Am J Obstetrics Gynecol* 2005; 192(2): 548-553. DOI: 10.1016/j.ajog.2004.08.028

[22] Cardenas VM, Mulla ZD, Ortiz M, Graham DY. Iron deficiency and Helicobacter pylori infection in the United States. *Am J Epidemiol* 2006; 163(2): 127-134. DOI: 10.1093/aje/kwj018

[23] Zhang ZF, Yang N, Zhao G, Zhu L, Zhu Y, Wang LX. Effect of Helicobacter pylori eradication on iron deficiency. *Chin Med J (Engl)* 2010; 123: 1924-1930.

[24] Yuan W, Li Yumin D, Yang L. Iron deficiency anemia in Helicobacter pylori infection: meta-analysis of randomized controlled trials. *Scand J Gastroenterol* 2010; 45 : 665-676 DOI: 10.3109/00365521003663670

[25] Muhsen K, Cohen D. Helicobacter pylori infection and iron stores: a systematic review and meta-analysis. *Helicobacter* 2008; 13: 323-340 DOI: 10.1111/j.1523-5378.2008.00617.x

[26] Huang X, Qu X, Yan W, Huang Y, Cai M, Hu B, Wu L, Lin H, Chen Z, Zhu C, Lu L, Sun X, Rong L, Jiang Y, Sun D, Zhong L, Xiong P. Iron deficiency anaemia can be improved after eradication of Helicobacter pylori. *Postgrad Med J* 2010; 86: 272-278. DOI: 10.1136/pgmj.2009.089987

[27] Qu XH, Huang XL, Xiong P, Zhu CY, Huang YL, Lu LG, Sun X, Rong L, Zhong L, Sun DY, Lin H, Cai MC, Chen ZW, Hu B, Wu LM, Jiang YB, Yan WL. Does Helicobacter pylori infec-tion play a role in iron deficiency anemia? A meta-analysis. *World J Gastroenterol* 2010; 16 : 886-896. DOI: 10.3748/wjg.v16.i7.886

[28] Muñoz Gómez M, Campos Garríguez A, García Erce JA, Ramírez Ramírez G. Fisiopathology of iron metabolism: diagnostic and therapeutic implications. *Nefrologia* 2005; 25(1): 9-19.

[29] Lombard M, Chua E, O'Toole P. Regulation of intestinal non-haem iron absorption. *Gut* 1997; 40: 435-439.

[30] McKie AT, Latunde-Dada GO, Miret S, McGregor JA, Anderson GJ, Vulpe C D, Wrigglesworth JM, Simpson RJ. Molecular evidence for the role of a ferric reductase in iron transport. *Biochem Soc Trans* 2002; 30: 722-724. DOI:10.1042/BST0300722

[31] Krishnamurthy P, Xie T, Schuetz JD. The role of transporters in cellular heme and porphyrin homeostasis. *Pharmacol Ther* 2007; 114(3): 345-358. DOI: 10.1016/j.pharmthera.2007.02.001

[32] Sargent PJ, Farnaud S, Evans RW. Structure/function overview ofproteins involved in iron storage and transport. *Curr Med Chem*2005; 12: 2683-2693. DOI. 10.2174/092986705774462969

[33] Siah CW, Ombiga J, Adams LA, Trinder D, Olynyk JK. Normal iron metabolism and the pathophysiology of iron overload disorders. *Clin Biochem Rev* 2006; 27(1): 5.

[34] Nemeth E, Ganz T. Hepcidin and iron-loading anemias. *Haematologica* 2006; 91(6): 727-732.

[35] Crichton RR, Danielsson BG, Geisser P. Iron metabolism: biologic and molecular aspects. Iron therapy with special emphasis on intravenous administration. 4th ed. Bremen: UNI-Med Verlag AG 2008, 14-24.

[36] Andrews NC. Forging a field: the golden age of iron biology. *Blood* 2008; 112(2): 219-230. DOI: 10.1182/blood-2007-12-077388

[37] Yip R, Limburg PJ, Ahlquist DA, Carpenter HA, O'Neill A, Kruse D, Stitham S, Gold BG, Gunter EW, Looker AC, Parkinson AJ, Nobmann ED, Petersen KM, Ellefson M, Schwartz S. Pervasive occult gastrointestinal bleeding in an Alaska native population with prevalent iron deficiency. Role of Helicobacter pylori gastritis. *JAMA* 1997; 277: 1135-1139. DOI: 10.1001/jama.1997.03540380049030

[38] Capurso G, Lahner E, Marcheggiano A, Caruana P, Carnuccio A, Bordi C, Delle Fave G, Annibale B. Involvement of the corporal mucosa and related changes in gastric acid secretion characterize patients with iron deficiency anaemia associated with Helicobacter pylori infection. *Aliment Pharmacol Ther* 2001; 15: 1753-1761. DOI: 10.1046/j.1365-2036.2001.01101.x

[39] Lee JH, Choe YH, Choi YO. The expression of iron repressible outer membrane proteins in Helicobacter pylori and its association with iron deficiency anemia. *Helicobacter* 2009; 14(1): 36-39. DOI: 10.1111/j.1523-5378.2009.00658.x

[40] Choe YH, Oh YJ, Lee NG, Imoto I, Adachi Y, Toyoda N, Gabazza EC. Lactoferrin sequestration and its contribution to iron-deficiency anemia in Helicobacter pylori-infected gastric mucosa. *J Gastroenterol Hepatol* 2003; 18: 980-985. DOI: 10.1046/j.1440-1746.2003.03098.x

[41] Van Leerdam ME. Epidemiology of acute upper gastrointestinal bleeding. *Best Practice Res Clin Gastroenterol* 2008; 22(2): 209-224. DOI: 10.1016/j.bpg.2007.10.011

[42] Kuipers EJ, Thijs JC, Festen HP. The prevalence of Helicobacter pylori in peptic ulcer disease. *Aliment Pharmacol Ther* 1994; 9: 59-69.

[43] Barkun AN, Bardou M, Kuipers EJ, Sung J, Hunt RH, Martel M, Sinclair P. International consensus recommendations on the management of patients with nonvariceal upper gastrointestinal bleeding. *Annals Internal Med* 2010; 152(2): 101-113. DOI: 10.7326/0003-4819-152-2-201001190-00009

[44] Gisbert JP, Khorrami S, Carballo F, Calvet X, Gené E, Dominguez-Muñoz E. Helicobacter pylori eradication therapy vs. antisecretory non-eradication therapy (with or without long-term maintenance antisecretory therapy) for the prevention of recurrent bleeding from peptic ulcer. *Cochrane Database System Rev* 2004; 19(6): 617-629. DOI: 10.1002/14651858.CD004062.pub2.

[45] Gisbert JP, Abraira V. Accuracy of Helicobacter pylori diagnostic tests in patients with bleeding peptic ulcer: a systematic review and meta-analysis. *Am J Gastroenterol* 2006; 101(4): 848-863. DOI: 10.1111/j.1572-0241.2006.00528.x

[46] Holster IL, Kuipers EJ. Management of acute nonvariceal upper gastrointestinal bleeding: current policies and future perspectives. *World J Gastroenterol: WJG* 2002; 18(11): 1202-1207. DOI: 10.3748/wjg.v18.i11.1202

[47] Kim SS, Ruiz VE, Carroll JD, Moss SF. Helicobacter pylori in the pathogenesis of gastric cancer and gastric lymphoma. *Cancer Lett* 2011; 305(2): 228-238. DOI: 10.1016/j.canlet.2010.07.014

[48] Suerbaum S, Michetti P. Helicobacter pylori infection. *N Engl J Med* 2002; 347: 1175-1186. DOI: 10.1056/NEJMra020542

[49] IARC Working Group. Schistosomes, liver flukes and Helicobacter pylori. IARC Working Group on the Evaluation of Carcinogenic Risks to Humans Lyon, 7–14 June 1994. *IARC Monogr Eval Carcinog Risks Hum* 1994; 61: 1-241.

[50] De Vries AC, Haringsma J, Kuipers EJ. The detection, surveillance and treatment of premalignant gastric lesions related to Helicobacter pyloriinfection. *Helicobacter* 2007; 12: 1-15. DOI: 10.1111/j.1523-5378.2007.00475.x

[51] Fock KM, Katelaris P, Sugano K, Ang TL, Hunt R, Talley NJ, Lam SK, Xiao SD, Tan HJ, Wu CY, Jung HC, Hoang BH, Kachintorn U, Goh KL, Chiba T, Rani AA. Second Asia-Pacific consensus guidelines for Helicobacter pylori infection. *J Gastroenterol Hepatol* 2009; 24: 1587-1600. DOI:10.1111/j.1440-1746.2009.05982.x

[52] Koike T, Ohara S, Sekine H, Iijima K, Abe Y, Kato K, Toyota T, Shimosegawa T. Helicobacter pylori infection prevents erosive reflux oesophagitis by decreasing gastric acid secretion. *Gut* 2001; 49(3): 330-334. DOI: 10.1136/gut.49.3.330

[53] Luzza F, Pensabene L, Imeneo M, Mancuso M, Contaldo A, Giancotti L, La Vecchia AM, Costa MC, Strisciuglio P, Docimo C, Pallone F, Guandalini S. Antral nodularity identifies children infected with Helicobacter pylori with higher grades of gastric inflammation. *Gastrointest Endosc* 2001; 53(1): 60-64.DOI:10.1067/mge.2001.111043

[54] Gisbert JP, Boixeda D, de Argila CM, Bermejo F, Redondo C, de Rafael L. Erosive duodenitis: prevalence of Helicobacter pylori infection and response to eradication therapy with omeprazole plus two antibiotics. *Eur J Gastroenterol Hepatol* 1997; 9(10): 957-962.

[55] Condrad ME, Umbreit JN, Moore EG. Iron absorption and transport. *Am J Med Sci* 1999; 318: 213-219. DOI:10.1097/00000441-199910000-00002

[56] Hines JD, Hoffbrand AV, Mollin DL. The haematologic complications following partial gastrectomy. A study of 292 patients. *Am J Med* 1967; 43: 555-569. DOI: 10.1016/0002-9343(67)90179-9

[57] Dickey W, Kenny BD, McMillan SA, Porter KG, McConnell JB. Gastric as well as duodenal biopsies may be useful in the investigation of iron deficiency anaemia. *Scand J Gastroenterol* 1997; 32: 469-472.

[58] Weinstein WM. Gastritis and gastropathies. In: Sleisinger MH, Fordtran JS, editors. *Gastrointestinal Disease*, 5th ed. Philadelphia: Saunders, 1993; pp. 545-571.

[59] Kuipers EJ, Pena AS, Festen HPM, Meuwissen SGM, Uyterlinde AM, Roosendaal R, Pals G, Nelis GF. Long-term sequelae of Helicobacter pylori gastritis. *Lancet* 1995; 345: 1525-1528. DOI: 10.1016/S0140-6736(95)91084-0

[60] Craanen ME, Blok P, Dekker W, Ferwerda J, Tytgat GN. Prevalence of subtypes of intestinal metaplasia in gastric antral mucosa. *Dig Dis Sci* 1991; 36(11): 1529-1536. DOI:10.1007/BF01296393

[61] Appelmelk BJ, Simoons-Smit I, Negrini R, Moran AP, Aspinall GO, Forte JG, De Vries T,Quan H, Verboom T, Maaskant JJ, Ghiara P, Kuipers EJ, Bloemena E, Tadema TM, Townsend RR, Tyagarajan K, Crothers Jr JM, Monteiro MA, Savio A, De Graaff J. Potential role of molecular mimicry between Helicobacter pylori lipopolysaccharide and host Lewis blood group antigens in autoimmunity. *Infect Immun* 1996; 64(6): 2031-2040.

[62] Malfertheiner P, Megraud F, O'Morain CA, Atherton J, Axon AT, Bazzoli F, Gensini GF, Gisbert JP, Graham DY, Rokkas T, El-Omar EM, Kuipers EJ. European Helico-

bacter Study Group. Management of Helicobacter pylori infection – the Maastricht IV/Florence consensus report. *Gut* 2012; 61(5): 646-664. DOI: 10.1136/gutjnl-2012-302084

[63] El-Omar EM, Oien K, El-Nujumi A, Gillen D, Wirz A, Dahill S, Williams C, Ardill JE, McColl KE. Helicobacter pylori infection and chronic gastric acid hyposecretion. *Gastroenterology* 1997; 113: 15-24. DOI: 10.1016/S0016-5085(97)70075-1

[64] Ruiz B, Rood JC, Fontham ETH, Malcom GT, Hunter FM, Sobhan M, Johnson WD, Correa P. Vitamin C concentration in gastric juice before and after anti Helicobacter pylori treatment. *Am J Gastroenterol* 1994; 4: 533-539.

[65] Banerjee S, Hawksby C, Miller S, Dahill S, Beattie AD, McColl KE. Effect of Helicobacter pyloriand its eradication on gastric juice ascorbic acid. *Gut* 1994;35:317-322. DOI: 10.1136/gut.35.3.317

[66] Koga T, Shimada Y, Sato K, Takahashi K, Kikuchi I, Okazaki Y, Miura T, Katsuta M, Iwata M. Contribution of ferrous iron to maintenance of the gastric colonization of Helicobacter pylori in miniature pigs. *Microbiol Res* 2002; 157(4): 323-330. DOI: 10.1078/0944-5013-00169

[67] Payne SM. Iron acquisition in microbial pathogenesis. *Trends Microbiol* 1993; 1(2): 66-69. DOI: 10.1016/0966-842X(93)90036-Q

[68] Andrews SC, Robinson AK, Rodriguez-Quinones F. Bacterial iron homeostasis. *FEMS Microbiol Rev* 2003; 27(2-3): 215-237. DOI: 10.1016/S0168-6445(03)00055-X

[69] Berg DE, Hoffman PS, Appelmelk BJ, Kusters JG. The Helicobacter pylori genome sequence: genetic factors for long life in the gastric mucosa. Trends Microbiol 1997; 5: 468-474. DOI: 10.1016/S0966-842X(97)01164-5

[70] Tomb JF, White O, Kerlavage AR, Clayton RA, Sutton GG, Fleischmann RD, Ketchum KA, Klenk HP, Gill S, Dougherty BA, Nelson K, Quackenbush J, Zhou L, Kirkness EF, Peterson S, Loftus B, Richardson D, Dodson R, Khalak HG, Glodek A, McKenney K, Fitzegerald LM, Lee N, Adams MD, Hickey EK, Berg DE, Gocayne JD, Utterback TR, Peterson JD, Kelley JM, Cotton MD, Weidman JM, Fujii C, Bowman C, Watthey L, Wallin E, Hayes WS, Borodovsky M, Karpk PD, Smith HO, Fraser CM, Venter JC. The complete genome sequence of the gastric pathogen Helicobacter pylori. *Nature* 1997; 388: 539-547.

[71] Alm RA, Ling LS, Moir DT, King BL, Brown ED, Doig PC, Smith DR, Noonan B, Guild BC, deJonge BL, Carmel G, Tummino PJ, Caruso A, Uria-Nickelsen M, Mills DM, Ives C, Gibson R, Merberg D, Mills SD, Jiang Q, Taylor DE, Vovis GF, Trust TJ. Genomic-sequence comparison of two unrelated isolates of the human gastric pathogen Helicobacter pylori. Nature 1999; 397: 176-180. DOI: 10.1038/16495

[72] van Vliet AHM, Bereswill S, Kusters JG. Ion metabolism and transport, In Mobley HLT, Mendz GL, and Hazell SL, editors, *Helicobacter Pylori*: Physiology and Genetics. ASM Press 2001, Washington, D.C.: pp. 193-206.

[73] Velayudhan J, Hughes NJ, McColm AA, Bagshaw J, Clayton CL, Andrews SC, Kelly DJ. Iron acquisition and virulence in Helicobacter pylori: a major role for FeoB, a high-affinity ferrous iron transporter. Mol Microbiol 2000; 37: 274-286. DOI:10.1046/j.1365-2958.2000.01987.x

[74] Worst DJ, Gerrits MM, Vandenbroucke-Grauls CM, Kusters JG. Helicobacter pylori ribBA-mediated riboflavin production is involved in iron acquisition. J Bacteriol 1998; 180: 1473-1479.

[75] van Vliet AHM, Stoof J, Vlasblom R, Wainwright SA, Hughes NJ, Kelly DJ, Bereswill S, Bijlsma JJ, Hoogenboezem T, Vandenbroucke-Grauls CM, Kist M, Kuipers EJ, Kusters JG. The role of the ferric uptake regulator (Fur) in regulation of Helicobacter pylori iron uptake. Helicobacter 2002; 7: 237-244. DOI:10.1046/j.1523-5378.2002.00088.x

[76] Guo Y, Guo G, Mao X, Zhang W, Xiao J, Tong W, Liu T, Xiao B, Liu X, Feng Y,Zou Q. Functional identification of HugZ, a heme oxygenase from Helicobacter pylori. *BMC Microbiol* 2008; 8(1): 226-237. DOI: 10.1186/1471-2180-8-226

[77] Wandersman C, Delepelaire P. Bacterial iron sources: from siderophores to hemophores. *Annu Rev Microbiol* 2004; 58: 611-647. DOI: 10.1146/annurev.micro.58.030603.123811

[78] Nakao K, Imoto I, Ikemura N, Shibata T, Takaji S, Taguchi Y, Misaki M, Yamauchi K, Yamazaki N. Relation of lactoferrin levels in gastric mucosa with Helicobacter pylori infection and with the degree of gastric inflammation. *Am J Gastroenterol* 1997; 92(6): 1005-1011.

[79] Bereswill S, Greiner S, van Vliet AHM, Waidner B, Fassbinder F, Schiltz E, Kusters JG, Kist M. Regulation of ferritin-mediated cytoplasmic iron storage by the ferric uptake regulator homolog (Fur) of Helicobacter pylori. J Bacteriol 2000; 182: 5948-5953. DOI: 10.1128/JB.182.21.5948-5953.2000

[80] Bereswill S, Waidner U, Odenbreit S, Lichte F, Fassbinder F, Bode G, Kist M. Structural, functional and mutational analysis of the pfr gene encoding a ferritin from Helicobacter pylori. Microbiology 1998; 144: 2505-2516.

[81] Doig P, Austin JW, Trust TJ. The Helicobacter pylori19.6-kilodalton protein is an iron-containing protein resembling ferritin. J Bacteriol 1993; 175: 557-560.

[82] Frazier BA, Pfeifer JD, Russell DG, Falk P, Olsen AN, Hammar M, Westblom TU, Normark SJ. Paracrystalline inclusions of a novel ferritin containing nonheme iron, produced by the human gastric pathogen Helicobacter pylori: evidence for a third class of ferritins. J Bacteriol 1993; 175: 966-972.

[83] Waidner B, Greiner S, Odenbreit S, Kavermann H, Velayudhan J, Stahler F, Guhl J, Bisse E, van Vliet AHM, Andrews SC, Kusters JG, Kelly DJ, Haas R, Kist M, Bereswill S.

Essential role of ferritin Pfr in Helicobacter pylori iron metabolism and gastric colonization. Infect Immun 2002; 70: 3923-3929. DOI: 10.1128/IAI.70.7.3923-3929.2002

[84] Evans DJ, Evans DG Jr, Takemura T, Nakano H, Lampert HC, Graham DY, Granger DN, Kvietys PR. Characterization of a Helicobacter pylori neutrophil-activating protein. Infect Immun 1995; 63: 2213-2220.

[85] Namavar F, Sparrius M, Veerman ECI, Appelmelk BJ, Vandenbroucke-Grauls CM. Neutrophil-activating protein mediates adhesion of Helicobacter pylori to sulfated carbohydrates on high-molecular-weight salivary mucin. Infect Immun 1998; 66: 444-447.

[86] Dundon WG, Polenghi A, Del Guidice G, Rappuoli R, Montecucco C. Neutrophil-activating protein (HP-NAP) versus ferritin (Pfr): comparison of synthesis in Helicobacter pylori. FEMS Microbiol Lett 2001; 199: 143-149. DOI:10.1111/j.1574-6968.2001.tb10665.x

[87] Tonello F, Dundon WG, Satin B, Molinari M, Tognon G, Grandi G, del Guicide G, Rappuoli R, Montecucco C. The Helicobacter pylori neutrophil-activating protein is an iron-binding protein with dodecameric structure. Mol Microbiol 1999; 34: 238-246. DOI:10.1046/j.1365-2958.1999.01584.x

[88] Cherian S, Forbes DA, Cook AG, Sanfiippo FM, Kemna EH, Swinkels DW, Burgner DP. An insight into the relationships between hepcidin, anemia, infections and inflammatory cytokines in pediatric refugees: a cross-sectional study. *PLoS One* 2008; 3: e4030. DOI:10.1371/journal.pone.0004030

[89] Schwarz P, Kübler JA, Strnad P, Müller K, Barth TF, Gerloff A, Feick P, Peyssonnaux C, Vaulont S, Adler G, Kulaksiz H. Hepcidin is localised in gastric parietal cells, regulates acid secretion and is induced by Helicobacter pylori infection. *Gut* 2012; 61(2): 193-201.DOI: 10.1136/gut.2011.241208

[90] Azab SF, Esh AM. Serum hepcidin levels in Helicobacter pylori-infected children with iron-deficiency anemia: a case-control study. *Ann Hematol* 2013; 92(11): 1477-1483. DOI: 10.1007/s00277-013-1813-2

[91] Ozkasap S, Yarali N, Isik P, Bay A, Kara A, Tunc B. The role of prohepcidin in anemia due to Helicobacter pylori infection. *Pediatr Hematol Oncol* 2013; 30(5): 425-431. DOI:10.3109/08880018.2013.783144

[92] Buommino E, Donnarumma G, Manente L, Filippis A, Silvestri F, Iaquinto S, Tufano MA, Luca A. The Helicobacter pylori protein HspB interferes with Nrf2/Keap1 pathway altering the antioxidant response of Ags cells. *Helicobacter* 2012; 17(6): 417-425. DOI:10.1111/j.1523-5378.2012.00973.x

[93] Gobert AP, Asim M, Piazuelo MB, Verriere T, Scull BP, de Sablet T, Glumac A, Lewis ND, Correa P, Peek RM Jr, Chaturvedi R, Wilson KT. Disruption of nitric oxide sig-

naling by Helicobacter pylori results in enhanced inflammation by inhibition of heme oxygenase-1. *J Immun* 2011; 187(10): 5370-5379. DOI:10.4049/jimmunol.1102111

[94] Bagnoli F, Buti L, Tompkins L, Covacci A, Amieva MR Helicobacter pylori CagA induces a transition from polarized to invasive phenotypes in MDCK cells. *Proc Natl Acad Sci U S A* 2005; 102: 16339-16344. DOI:10.1073/pnas.0502598102

[95] Tan S, Noto JM, Romero-Gallo J, Peek RM Jr, Amieva MR. Helicobacter pylori perturbs iron trafficking in the epithelium to grow on the cell surface. *PLoS Pathog* 2011;7(5): e1002050. DOI: 10.1371/journal.ppat.1002050

[96] Capurso G, Martino M, Grossi C, Annibale B, Delle Fave G. Hypersecretory duodenal ulcer and Helicobacter pylori infection: a four-year follow-up study. *Dig Liv Dis* 2000; 32: 119-124. DOI: 10.1016/S1590-8658(00)80397-7

[97] Sipponen P, Kekki M, Seppala K, Siurala M. The relationship between chronic gastritis and gastric acid secretion. *Aliment Pharmacol Ther* 1996; 10: 103-118. DOI: 10.1046/j.1365-2036.1996.22164011.x

[98] Furuta T, Baba S, Takashima M, Futami H, Arai H, Kajimura M, Hanai H, Kaneko E. Effect of Helicobacter pylori infection on gastric juice pH. *Scand J Gastroenterol* 1998; 33: 357-363. DOI: 10.1080/00365529850170973

[99] Ciacci C, Sabbatini F, Cavallaro R, Castiglione F, Di Bella S, Iovino P, Palumbo A, Tortora R, Amoruso D, Mazzacca G. Helicobacter pylori impairs iron absorption in infected individuals. *Dig Liver Dis* 2004;36(7): 455-460. DOI: 10.1016/j.dld.2004.02.008

[100] Ge R, Sun X. Iron trafficking system in Helicobacter pylori. *Biometals* 2012; 25(2): 247-258. DOI: 10.1007/s10534-011-9512-9518

[101] Baysoy G, Ertem D, Ademoglu E, Kotiloglu E, Keskin S, Pehlivanoglu E. Gastric histopathology, iron status and iron deficiency anemia in children with Helicobacter pylori infection. *J Pediatr Gastroenterol Nutr* 2004; 38(2): 146-151. DOI: 10.1097/00005176-200402000-00008

[102] Cardenas VM, Prieto-Jimenez CA, Mulla ZD, Rivera JO, Dominguez DC, Graham DY, Ortiz M. Helicobacter pylori eradication and change in markers of iron stores among non–iron-deficient children in El Paso, Texas: an etiologic intervention study. *J Pediatr Gastroenterol Nutr* 2011; 52(3): 326-332. DOI: 10.1097/MPG.0b013e3182054123

[103] Zagari RM, Romano M, Ojetti V, Stockbrugger R, Gullini S, Annibale B, Farinati F, Ierardi E, Maconi G, Rugge M, Calabrese C, Di Mario F, Luzza F, Pretolani S, Savio A, Gasbarrini G, Caselli M. Guidelines for the management of Helicobacter pylori infection in Italy: The III Working Group Consensus Report 2015. *Dig Liver Dis* 2015; 47(11): 903-912. DOI:10.1016/j.dld.2015.06.010

[104] Campuzano-Maya G. Hematologic manifestations of Helicobacter pylori infection. *World J Gastroenterol: WJG* 2014; 20(36): 12818-12838 DOI: 10.3748/wjg.v20.i36.12818

[105] Hershko C, Skikne B. Pathogenesis and management of iron deficiency anemia: emerging role of celiac disease, helicobacter pylori, and autoimmune gastritis. *Sem Hematol WB* Saunders 2009; 46(4): 339-350. DOI: 10.1053/j.seminhematol.2009.06.002

[106] Habib HSA, Murad HAS, Amir EM, Halawa TF. Effect of sequential versus standard Helicobacter pylori eradication therapy on the associated iron deficiency anemia in children. *Ind J Pharmacol* 2013; 45(5): 470-473. DOI: 10.4103/0253-7613.117757

Section 4

# Helicobacter pylori and Metabolic Disorders

Chapter 6

# *Helicobacter pylori* Infection and Diabetes Mellitus

Saeda Haj, Michal Raviv and Khitam Muhsen

Additional information is available at the end of the chapter

http://dx.doi.org/10.5772/63826

**Abstract**

*Helicobacter pylori* colonizes the stomach and causes chronic gastritis, which most often remains asymptomatic. However, in a small proportion of infected persons, it causes peptic ulcers and gastric cancer. We reviewed recent evidence of the association between *H. pylori* infection and diabetes mellitus (DM). Numerous studies have shown a positive association between *H. pylori* infection and DM, however, findings are still conflicting. Such a link is biologically plausible, given the importance of the stomach in the homeostasis of systems outside the digestive tract; however, the mechanisms by which *H. pylori* might affect the risk of DM are not clear. Current knowledge indicates that *H. pylori* infection can affect the regulation of ghrelin and leptin, two hormones that play central roles in energy homeostasis in humans. Yet, methodological limitations are present in studies that addressed the relationships of *H. pylori* infection with DM and with possible risk factors for DM, including inadequate control of confounders. The important question of whether *H. pylori* eradication might be beneficial for glycemic control in diabetic patients is still unresolved. Future well-designed studies are needed to address these research questions, which are of clinical and great public health significance.

**Keywords:** Helicobacter pylori, diabetes mellitus, epidemiology

## 1. Introduction

*Helicobacter pylori* is a gram-negative bacterium that colonizes the stomach and causes persistent infection. The infection is typically acquired in the first few years of life [1–3]. The associated risk factors of *H. pylori* infection include living in crowded households, low socioeconomic conditions and infected family members [4–6]. The infection is common worldwide with highest prevalence rates reaching 80–90% in developing countries and underprivileged communities [7], while a much lower prevalence of 20–50% is recorded in developed countries [7].

*H. pylori* infection has two phases: an acute phase and a chronic course. Acute *H. pylori* infection is rarely diagnosed. Following establishment of the infection, chronic gastritis develops; however, most infected people remain asymptomatic and only 10–20% of them develop peptic disease during their lifetime [7]. *H. pylori* causes gastric and duodenal ulcers, and in rare occasions distal gastric cancer and mucosa-associated lymphoid tissue (MALT) lymphoma [7]. These diseases are the main indications to test and treat *H. pylori* infection [8], in addition to unexplained iron deficiency anemia (IDA) and idiopathic thrombocytopenic purpura [8]. Although *H. pylori* infection is acquired in childhood, peptic ulcer disease typically occurs in adulthood.

Following *H. pylori* colonization, rigorous local and systemic immune responses develop. However, these do not clear the infection but rather contribute to the damage of the gastric mucosa [7, 9, 10]. *H. pylori* simulates the innate immune response, as well as humoral and cell-mediated immune responses [9, 10]. The predominant human T cell response is the T-helper 1 mediated response, which is associated with releasing proinflammatory cytokines and activation of phagocytes [9, 10]. *H. pylori* also induces Th2 and T-regulatory (Tregs) responses [9, 10]. The importance of Treg response is in both controlling inflammation and promoting the persistence of the infection [9, 10].

*H. pylori*-associated gastric pathology develops over time in a progressive manner [11–13], and the damage to gastric mucosa can be observed even in asymptomatic persons [14]. Today it is clear that host (e.g., age, genetic susceptibility), agent (virulence antigens) and environment-related factors are important in the development of *H. pylori*-associated gastroduodenal diseases [9]. For example, host genetic polymorphisms that lead to increased release of proinflammatory cytokines are associated with increased gastric cancer risk [9]. Pathogenesis is dependent on a Th1-acquired immune response and on hormonal changes including hypergastrinemia [9]. Regarding pathogen virulence factors, most *H. pylori* strains carry the *cag* pathogenicity island that encodes for a type IV secretory apparatus, which allows translocation of cytotoxin-associated gene A (CagA) protein into the host cell. This, together with the vacuolating cytotoxin (VacA), plays a major role in the pathogenesis of gastroduodenal diseases [7, 9, 15–17]. Novel *H. pylori* antigens have been identified recently [18], some of which were found to be associated with atrophic gastritis and gastric cancer risk such as GroEL [18], Helicobacter cysteine-rich protein (HcpC) [19], outer membrane protein (Omp) and others [20, 21].

Several studies have shown associations between *H. pylori* infection and various extragastric diseases [22]. *H. pylori* infection was positively linked with adulthood chronic diseases such as cardiovascular disease [23–25], dementia [26–28], insulin resistance and diabetes mellitus (DM) [22, 29, 30]. The mechanisms of such associations are not fully understood, and it is not clear whether such associations are causal or not. This chapter will focus on the association between *H. pylori* infection and DM.

## 2. *H. pylori* infection, changes in gastric physiology and metabolic hemostasis

Although the role of *H. pylori* infection in the pathogenesis of gastroduodenal diseases [7, 9, 17, 31] is well established, its impeding effects on metabolic homeostasis and DM are not clear.

The stomach plays a major role in the homeostasis of systems outside the digestive tract. Therefore, the link between *H. pylori*-chronic gastritis and metabolic homeostasis and DM seems biologically plausible.

*H. pylori*-induced inflammation and its severity affect gastric physiology. For example, *H. pylori* leads to hormonal changes in the stomach, such as reduced production of somatostatin and hypergastrinemia [9]. *H. pylori*-gastritis also alters the secretion of gastric acid [32, 33]; increased secretion of gastric acid is associated with antral-predominant phenotype and increased risk of duodenal ulcers [9, 10]. *H. pylori* infection can reduce gastric acid production, and this is typically associated with corpus-predominant gastritis and increased likelihood of gastric ulcer and gastric adenocarcinoma [9, 10]. Moreover, *H. pylori* infection is associated with reduced gastric ascorbic acid levels [34]. *H. pylori* affects the levels of pepsinogen (PG) I and PGII; proenzymes of the digestive enzyme pepsin. PGI is secreted from cells in the corpus and PGII is also secreted from cells in the antrum and duodenum [35, 36]. About 1% of PGs can be found in the serum. Serum PGI and PGII are increased in *H. pylori* infected vs. uninfected individuals, and higher levels are found in more severe gastritis. As the severity of gastritis progresses and corpus atrophic lesions appear, the PGI level decreases, while the PGII level remains stable; the result is a decrease in the PGI:PGII ratio [37, 38]. These markers have clinical significance, and they predict various gastric pathologies [16, 37–40].

In addition, *H. pylori* infection can affect the regulation of ghrelin and leptin [41–47], two hormones that play central roles in energy homeostasis [48]. Ghrelin reduces energy expenditure and promotes weight gain [48–50], while leptin decreases appetite and increases energy expenditure [48]. Both hormones are secreted by the epithelial cells in the stomach [48, 51]. The relationship between *H. pylori* and these hormones appears to be complex. While several studies reported no association between *H. pylori* infection and circulating leptin [43, 45, 46, 52–54] and ghrelin levels [45, 52, 54], others found lower levels of one or the two hormones in *H. pylori* infected vs. uninfected individuals [41, 42, 44]. There also appears to be differences in gastric mucosa levels of these hormones, according to *H. pylori* infection [41, 42, 47, 52–54]. Moreover, *H. pylori* eradication seems to affect these hormones as well [41, 43, 45, 47, 52] (Table 1).

| **Study** | **Exposure** | **Ghrelin** | | **Leptin** | |
|---|---|---|---|---|---|
| | | **Circulating levels** | **Gastric mucosa levels** | **Circulating levels** | **Gastric mucosa levels** |
| Isomoto et al. [44] | *H. pylori* infection | ↓ | ↓ | ND | ND |
| | *H. pylori* eradication | NS | NS | ND | ND |
| Chuang et al. [46] | *H. pylori* infection | Males: ↓<br>Females: NS | ND | NS | ND |
| Jun et al. [52] | *H. pylori* infection | NS | NS | NS | ↑ |
| Nishi et al. [53] | *H. pylori* infection | ND | ND | NS | ↑ |

| Study | Exposure | Ghrelin | | Leptin | |
|---|---|---|---|---|---|
| | | Circulating levels | Gastric mucosa levels | Circulating levels | Gastric mucosa levels |
| | *H. pylori* eradication | ND | ND | NS | |
| Francois et al. [45] | *H. pylori* infection | NS | ND | NS | ND |
| | *H. pylori* eradication | Pre-meal: NS<br>Post meal: ↑ | ND | ↑ | ND |
| Azuma et al. [47] | *H. pylori* infection | ND | ND | | ↑ |
| | *H. pylori* eradication | ND | ND | NS | ↓ |
| Jang et al. [54] | *H. pylori* eradication | NS | ↑ | NS | ND |
| Roper et al. [41] | *H. pylori* infection | NS | Fundic: NS<br>Antral: NS<br>Gastric juice: ↑ | ↓ | Fundic: NS<br>Antral: ↓ |
| Breidert et al. [43] | *H. pylori* infection | ND | ND | NS | Antrum: NS<br>Corpus: ↑ |

NS, no significant difference; ND, not determined;, ↑ increase;, ↓ decrease.

**Table 1.** Selected studies that addressed associations of *H. pylori* infection and *H. pylori* eradication with ghrelin and leptin levels

Altogether, these studies suggest that *H. pylori* can alter gastric physiology, which can in turn affect metabolic homeostasis and the risk of DM.

## 3. *H. pylori* infection and diabetes mellitus

DM refers to a group of metabolic disorders that manifest with hyperglycemia. DM is classified based on the pathogenic course that results in hyperglycemia, with two broad categories designated as type 1 DM (T1DM) and type 2 DM (T2DM). T1DM is the result of interaction among genetic, environmental and immunological factors that eventually leads to destruction of beta cells in the pancreas and complete or near-complete insulin deficiency. T2DM consists of various disorders with variable levels of insulin resistance, impaired insulin secretion and increased glucose production. T1DM usually occurs in childhood and adolescence, and comprises 5–10% of all DM cases [55]. T2DM typically develops in adulthood and is responsible for the majority (90–95%) of DM cases [55].

DM is a major public health problem [56–60], causing an enormous burden to patients and their families, as well as to health care systems. The prevalence of T2DM is increasing globally

[56–60] due to increases in life expectancy and obesity [56, 58]. It is estimated that 240 million people have T2DM, and that in 2025 about 380 million will have the disease, while 418 million will have impaired glucose tolerance (IGT) [56]. The burden of DM is amplified given its significant macro and microvascular complications (such as cardiovascular disease, kidney disease), in addition to peripheral neuropathy [55].

There are well-established risk factors for T2DM [61–67], including sociodemographic factors [64, 68, 69], lifestyle factors (e.g., obesity, physical inactivity, poor diet [61–67]) and high glucose levels reflecting IGT [65, 66]. Changes in diet (i.e., higher consumption of whole grain products and exchanging unsaturated fat for saturated fat), and in particular physical activity and avoidance of obesity, can prevent T2DM through changes in body fat and other mechanisms [61, 67, 70–72]. These may reduce the incidence of DM by 28–59% [72]. Such interventions are also important for better control of diabetes [70, 73]. Current evidence suggests that there must be additional factors besides lifestyle that contribute to the occurrence of DM.

In addition to the association mentioned above, between *H. pylori* infection and ghrelin and leptin [41, 45, 74–80], associations have been reported of *H. pylori* infection with glycated hemoglobin levels (Hb1Ac) [81], as well as with disturbances in metabolic homeostasis including insulin resistance; the latter according to a recent literature review and a systematic review [22, 82]. These findings support the postulation that *H. pylori* infection may be involved in the etiology of the emerging pandemic of obesity and DM, and in diabetes-related complications.

Associations of *H. pylori* infection with DM incidence [30, 83, 85] have been reported. Recent meta-analyses showed a significant 1.7 to 2-fold higher prevalence of *H. pylori* infection in persons with T2DM vs. non-diabetic individuals [84, 85]. In some of the studies that reported a positive association between *H. pylori* infection and DM [30, 86–88], the association became non-statistically significant after adjustment for potential confounders such as age and socioeconomic status [87, 88]. Other studies reported no significant association between *H. pylori* and DM [89–92], or a significant association only in persons with BMI>25 [81] (Table 2). Several studies did not control adequately for socioeconomic status and for traditional risk factors of DM, such as obesity and physical inactivity. Furthermore, most of the evidence is based on small-scale hospital-based case–control studies, in which the source population, selection of control population and representativeness of the sample were not fully described. For these reasons, inference and generalizability of findings from such studies should be done with caution. On the other hand, recent well-designed studies show convincing evidence of the potential involvement of *H. pylori* infection in the occurrence of DM, and possibly in IGT. A large population-based follow-up investigation of elderly persons has demonstrated a significant two-fold increased risk of DM in *H. pylori* infected vs. uninfected persons, even after controlling for possible confounders, while such an association was not observed for other pathogens [30]. A large well-designed and thoroughly analyzed survey that utilized nationwide data (*N*~13,000) from the United States indicated no significant association between *H. pylori* infection and self-reported diabetes. However, among individuals with BMI>25 kg/m$^2$ who were assessed in the 1999–2000 National Health & Nutrition Examination Survey (NHANES), DM was more prevalent among those who were *H. pylori* seropositive than those who were *H. pylori*-seronegative[81] (Table 2). Moreover, that study showed that *H. pylori* infected persons, especially those infected with CagA strains, had significantly elevated mean HbA1c levels compared with those who were *H. pylori* seronegative [81].

| Study | Study population | Study design | *Hp detection* | Outcome | Findings | Adjusting for confounders |
|---|---|---|---|---|---|---|
| Jeon et al. [30] California | *N*=782 diabetes free individuals at baseline Age >60 years | Prospective cohort | Serum IgG by ELISA | DM | Adjusted HR 2.69 (95% CI: 1.10–6.60) | Sex, education, smoking, cholesterol, DBP, HSV-1 |
| Hsieh et al. [86] Taiwan | *N*=903 *Hp* infected patients aged 57.16±11.64 years<br>*N*=1167 uninfected patients aged 56.57±13.34 years | Cross-sectional | Gastric biopsy: culture, histology and rapid urease test | T2DM | OR 1.67 (95% CI: 1.19–2.35) | |
| Chen and Blaser [81] USA | Data from NHANES III *N*=7417 age ≥18 years<br>NHANES 1999–2000 *N*=6072 age ≥3 years | Cross-sectional | Serum IgG by ELISA | DM | NHANES 1999–2000: Adjusted OR: 1.30 (95% CI: 0.94–1.80)<br>BMI>25 OR (1.43; 95% CI: 1.00–2.03)<br>NHANES III: Adjusted OR: 0.99 (95% CI: 0.80–1.23) | Age, sex, race, BMI, smoking, education |
| El-Eshmawy et al. [111] Egypt | *N*=162 T1DM patients aged 19.35±2.6 years<br>*N*=80 healthy subjects aged 19.76±2.76 years | Case-control | Serum IgG and IgA by ELISA | T1DM | OR 3.67 (95% CI: 2.07–6.55) | Matching by age, sex, SES |
| Longo-Mbenza et al. [91] Democratic Republic of the Congo | *N*=128 patients with *Hp* infection aged 53.4±12.9 years<br>*N*=77 uninfected patients aged 52.5±16.6 years | Prospective cohort Follow-up 9.6±0.8 years | Serum IgG by ELISA | DM | OR: 0.97 (95% CI: 0.35–2.86) | |
| Xia et al. [89] Australia | *N*=49 T1DM and *N*=380 T2DM (aged 60.7±13.3 years)<br>*N*=170 non-diabetic controls aged 60.4± 11.3 years | Case-control | Serum IgG by ELISA | T1DM T2DM | Overall 0.94 (95% CI: 0.65–1.39)<br>T2DM: OR: 1.03 (95% CI: 0.71–1.52)<br>T1DM: OR: 0.40 (95% CI: 0.15–0.94) | |

| Study | Study population | Study design | *Hp detection* | Outcome | Findings | Adjusting for confounders |
|---|---|---|---|---|---|---|
| Demir et al. [90] Turkey | *N*=141 T2DM patients aged 52±8.2 years *N*=142 non-diabetic subjects aged 51±9.3 years | Case-control | Gastric biopsy: rapid urease test and histology | T2DM | OR: 1.15 (95% CI: 0.71–1.85) | |
| Colombo et al. [112] Italy | *N*=138 T1DM patients aged 12.0±3.4 years *N*=138 controls aged 12.2±2.0 years | Case-control | Serum IgG and IgA by ELISA | T1DM | OR: 0.87 (95% CI: 0.52–1.46) | Matching by age |
| Cenerelli et al. [92] Italy | *N*=30 T2DM patients aged 55.7±9.7 years *N*=43 controls aged 51.2±11.3 years | Case-control | UBT | T2DM | OR: 1.06 (95% CI: 0.41–2.76) | |
| Dore et al. [87] | *N*=145 T1DM and *N*=240 T2DM *N*=506 controls (ages 12–75 years) | Case-control | Serum IgG by ELISA | T1DM T2DM | T1DM: 0.59 (95%CI: 0.40–0.87) T2DM: 2.08 (95%CI: 1.52–2.85) | In stratified analysis by age group, SES, the differences were not significant |
| Lutsey et al. [88] | *N*= 1000 ages 45–84 years | Cross-sectional | Serum IgG by ELISA | DM | Crude OR: 1.65 (95%CI: 1.16–2.34) Adjusted OR: 1.12 (0.78–1.62) | Age, sex, rate, education and site |

BMI, body mass index; CI, confidence intervals; DM, diabetes mellitus; DBP, diastolic blood pressure; ELISA, enzyme-linked immunosorbent assay; *Hp*, *Helicobacter pylori*; HR, hazard ratio; HSV-1, *Herpes simplex virus* 1; IgA, immunoglobulin A; IgG, immunoglobulin G; NHANES, National Health & Nutrition Examination Survey; OR, odd ratio: SES, socioeconomic status; T1DM, type 1 diabetes mellitus; T2DM, type 2 diabetes mellitus; UBT, urea breath test.

**Table 2.** Selected epidemiological studies that examined an association between *H. pylori* infection and diabetes mellitus

## 4. *H. pylori* infection and glycemic control among diabetic patients

Given the observed associations between *H. pylori* infection and various metabolic and glycemic measures, the question arises of whether *H. pylori* infection and/or *H. pylori* eradication can affect glycemic control in diabetic patients. If indeed *H. pylori* infection plays a role in glycemic control, *H. pylori* eradication might be beneficial to diabetic patients. A recent meta-analysis that included 14 observational studies involving 1781 diabetic patients (both T1DM and T2DM) showed no significant difference in mean HbA1c values among *H. pylori* infected individuals compared with those uninfected; mean difference 0.19% (95% CI: −0.18 to 0.46),

(Pv=0.16) [93]. In contrast, another meta-analysis involving 11 studies and 513 patients reported significantly higher HbA1c values among *H. pylori*-infected diabetic persons than among uninfected ones: weighted mean difference 0.43 (95% CI: 0.07–0.79), (Pv=0.02) [94]. The discrepancy in results between the two meta-analyses can be explained by differences in their criteria of study selection, which determined the number and quality of the studies analyzed.

| Study | Study population | *H. pylori* infection | Intervention | Outcome | Findings | Adjusting for confounders |
|---|---|---|---|---|---|---|
| **T2DM** | | | | | | |
| Zojaji et al. [95] Iran | *Hp* positive T2DM patients ($N$=85). Mean age 52.3 ±4.7 yrs, 31.8% males | Serum IgG antibodies by ELISA | OCA for 14 d. | HbA1c, FPG | Mean HbA1c levels before successful treatment were 8.7±1.1% and 3 m. after treatment were 8.3±0.9% ($P$<0.001)<br>FPG before successful treatment were 145±22 mg/dl and 3 m. after treatment were 133±18 mg/dl (NS)<br>No significant change in HbA1c was found before and after therapy among patients with no successful *Hp* eradication | None |

http://dx.doi.org/10.5772/63826

| | | | | | | |
|---|---|---|---|---|---|---|
| Vafaeimanes et al. [97]<br>Iran | *N*=191 *Hp* positive patients aged 55.6±9.8 yrs, 53.9% males<br>T2DM patients non-insulin users (*N*=93) and non-diabetic patients (*N*=98) with upper GI symptoms | Gastroscopy and biopsy: histology | Quadruple therapy for 14 d. (*N*= 96; 47 diabetic and 49 non-diabetic patients): OMAB<br>Triple therapy for 14 d. (*N*=95; 46 diabetic and 49 non-diabetic patients): OCA | HbA1c, FPG | *Hp* eradication was successful in 63% of T2DM patients vs. 87.7% in non-diabetic patients who received OCA therapy ($P$=0.017) and 38.2 vs. 55.1%, respectively ($P$< 0.001) in those who received OMAB<br>Decrease in HbA1c level 3 and 6 m after treatment was 0.23±0.91% vs. 0.25±0.85% and 0.19±0.85% vs. 0.20±0.91% in T2DM patients who had successful *Hp* eradication vs. no eradication, respectively (NS) | Age and sex-matching between diabetic and non-diabetic patients |

| | | | | | |
|---|---|---|---|---|---|
| | | | | | Decrease in FPG level 3 and 6 m. after treatment was 10.9±12.1 mg/dl vs. 9.5±14.3 mg/dl and 8.9±16.8 mg/dl vs. 9.4±15.6 mg/dl in T2DM patients who had successful *Hp* eradication vs. no eradication, respectively (NS) |
| Wada et al. [96]<br><br>Japan | T2DM patients (*N*=72) who received *Hp* eradication therapy. Mean age 63.7 ±1.1 yrs, 76.4% males | Gastric biopsy | AC plus lansoprazole (*N*=65) or Omeprazole (*N*=2), or rabeprazole (*N*=5) for 7 d. | HbA1c | HbA1c levels did not show significant change after therapy 6.9% ±0.1% 3 m. before to 7.0 ±0.1% 3 m. after (*P*=0.3), 7.0 ±0.1% after 6 m. (*P*=0.3) |
| Akanuma et al. [98]<br><br>Japan | T2DM *Hp* infected patients (*N*=174) aged 65±7 yrs, 83.9% males without GI complications who had successful *Hp* eradication therapy | Gastroscopy biopsy:<br><br>Culture, histology,, rapid urease test serum IgG antibodies<br><br>UBT | First-line treatment: LR or OCA (*N*=119)<br><br>Patients with penicillin allergy: LCM (*N*=3)<br><br>Quadruple therapy: LACM (*N*=24)<br><br>Second-line therapy: lansoprazole or | HbA1c | Overall, no significant changes in mean HbA1c values were observed 1 year before and after *Hp* eradication (*P*=0.07)<br><br>Among patients with uncontrolled diabetes (*N*=76), HbA1c levels decreased |

| | | | | | | |
|---|---|---|---|---|---|---|
| | | | RAM (*N*=28)<br><br>Regimens were given for 7 d. | | significantly between baseline and post *Hp* eradication (*P*=0.08): 8.22±0.92% at baseline 8.08 ±1.1% 3 m.<br><br>7.95 ±1.2% 6 m.<br><br>8.06 ±1.1% 9 m.<br><br>7.99 ±0.99% 12 m.<br><br>Among patients with controlled diabetes (*N*=98), HbA1c levels increased between baseline and post-*Hp* eradication (*P*=0.41): 6.77±0.4% at baseline6 .88 ±0.6% 3 m.<br><br>6.97 ±0.6% 6 m.<br><br>7.00 ±0.6% 9 m.<br><br>7.01 ±0.6% 12 m. | |
| **T1DM** | | | | | | |
| Candelli et al. [99]<br><br>Italy | T1DM patients aged 13.6±4.6 yrs, 51.7% males infected with *Hp* | UBT | ACR for 7 d. | HbA1c | No difference in HbA1c level was observed between *Hp* infected and | Sex, age, family income, BMI |

| | | | | | | |
|---|---|---|---|---|---|---|
| | (*N*=29) and uninfected T1DM patients aged 13.1±4.2 yrs, 51.7% males (*N*=29) | | | | uninfected patients.<br><br>8.25±1.06% vs. 8.4±1.7% (NS)<br><br>No difference in HbA1c level was observed in patients before and 6 m. after eradication 8.2±1% vs. 8.3±1% (NS) nor between *Hp* infected patients and uninfected ones 6 m after the evaluation of *Hp* status | |
| Begue et al. [100]<br><br>Louisiana | T1DM patients aged 7–17 yrs with asymptomatic *Hp* infection (*N*=8) and uninfected T1DM patients aged 6–18 (*N*=16) | Serum IgG antibodies, UBT | OCM for 14 d. | HbA1c | HbA1c values were higher among T1DM *Hp* infected patients than T1DM uninfected patients at the beginning of the study (median, 13.6% and 11.0%, respectively; $P$=0.07)<br><br>After treatment, T1DM *Hp*-infected patients had a steady decrease in HbA1c level (slope = −0.10), whereas uninfected T1DM patients had a slightly increasing trend (slope= +0.03) ($P$= 0.05) | Age, race, BMI, diabetes duration and compliance with clinical appointments |

| | | | | | |
|---|---|---|---|---|---|
| | | | | | After 2 yrs, HbA1c values were similar in *Hp* infected and uninfected patients (median: 11.7 and 11.4%, respectively; $P = 0.69$) |
| de Luis et al. [101] Spain | *Hp*-infected T1DM patients ($N$=13) aged 44.9±15.5 yrs, 30.77% males | Serum IgG antibodies, UBT, gastric biopsy | First-line therapy OCA for 10 d. In persistent infection: retreatment adding bismuth for 10 d. | HbA1c | HbA1c levels before and 6 m after *Hp* eradication were 7.%±1.7%vs. 7.5±0.6% in patients free of gastritis ($N$=9) and 7.1±1.1% vs. 6.8±1.4% in patients with gastritis ($N$=4). All NS |

A, amoxicillin; B, bismuth; BMI, body mass index; C, clarithromycin; d, days; ELISA, enzyme linked immunosorbent assay; FPG, fasting plasma glucose; GI, gastrointestinal; HbA1c, glycosylated hemoglobin; *Hp*, *Helicobacter pylori*; IgG, immunoglobulin G; L, lansoprazole; m, months; NS, not significant; O, omeprazole; OCA, omeprazole 20 mg and clarithromycin 500 mg and amoxicillin 1 g each twice a day; OMAB, omeprazole 20 mg and metronidazole 500 mg and amoxicillin 1 g and bismuth subcitrate 240 mg, each twice a day; PU, peptic ulcer; R, rabeprazole; SES, socioeconomic status; T1DM, type 1 diabetes mellitus; T2DM, type 2 diabetes mellitus; UBT, urea breath test; yrs, years.

**Table 3.** *Helicobacter pylori* eradication and glycemic control in diabetic patients

The question of whether *H. pylori* eradication can improve glycemic control was assessed in a limited number of observational studies, most of them were small scale [95–101] (Table 3). Findings from these studies were conflicting, ranging from no difference, to small non-significant or borderline improvements from baseline to up to 2-years after eradication [95–101] and to a significant decrease from baseline, in HbA1c at 3 months after *H. pylori* eradication [95]. A pooled analysis of two studies that compared mean differences in HbA1c between diabetic individuals who had undergone successful *H. pylori* eradication and those whose *H. pylori* eradication therapy had failed, showed no significant difference between the groups [94]. The optimal study design to examine the effect of *H. pylori* eradication therapy on glycemic control is a randomized controlled trial with intention-to-treat analysis, in which diabetic patients are assigned to either an *H. pylori* eradication group or a placebo control group. However, to-date such trials are lacking, and the current evidence is based on observational studies, which are evidently prone to biases and confounders. Therefore, the question of whether *H. pylori* infection affects glycemic control in diabetic patients remains unresolved.

## 5. *H. pylori* infection and metabolic syndrome

Metabolic syndrome is a cluster of metabolic risk factors that are associated with increased risk for atherosclerotic cardiovascular disease, T2DM and their complications. These factors include atherogenic dyslipidemia (elevated triglycerides and apolipoprotein B, increases small low-density lipoproteins [LDL], and low concentration of high-density lipoproteins [HDL]), elevated blood pressure and elevated fasting glucose levels known as impaired fasting glucose (IFG) or prediabetes [102, 103], which lead to a prothrombotic and proinflammatory state. The main risk factors for metabolic syndrome include obesity, mainly abdominal obesity and insulin resistance [103], as well as aging, physical inactivity and diet rich with saturated fat and cholesterol [103].

Recent studies have tested the hypothesis of a positive association between *H. pylori* and metabolic syndrome [22, 104–106]. While the underlying mechanisms remain to be determined, the inflammatory response to infection and secretion of cytokines such as tumor necrosis factor alpha (TNF-$\alpha$) and interleukin-1 (IL-1), IL-6 and IL-8 likely play a role in the postulated association. Additionally, *H. pylori*-induced atrophic gastritis, which develops with aging, reduces the levels of vitamin B12 and folate, which increase homocysteine levels, a known risk factor for insulin resistance [104].

The evidence from epidemiological studies on the association between *H. pylori* infection and metabolic syndrome has been evolving over the past few years.

A recent large cross-sectional study conducted among 3578 persons aged 18–64 years from Taiwan has demonstrated that *H. pylori* infected persons (according to urea breath test [UBT]) had a significantly increased prevalence of metabolic syndrome than uninfected persons; 12.4 vs. 7.4% (Pv<0.001) in men and 7.4 vs. 2.5% in women (Pv<0.001) [105]. In this study, metabolic syndrome was defined based on National Cholesterol Education Program (NCEP) Adult Treatment Panel (ATP) III Criteria, which were adjusted to the Taiwanese population [105].

The observed positive associations between *H. pylori* infection and metabolic syndrome were attenuated in multivariable analyses, while adjusting for confounders such as age, smoking and alcohol drinking; adjusted odds ratio (OR) 1.91 (95% CI: 1.03–3.53) in women, while in men the association was not statistically significant: adjusted OR: 1.38 (95% CI: 0.97–1.95) [105].

A population-based study conducted among adults aged 25 years or over in Iran also reported a 1.5-fold significantly increased prevalence of metabolic syndrome (according to NCEP-ATP-III criteria) among *H. pylori* (based on serum IgG detection) infected men and women compared with uninfected ones [107]. The same study reported positive associations in relation to exposure to other infectious agents as well such as *Chlamydia pneumoniae, Herpes simplex virus 1* (HSV-1) and *Cytomegalovirus* (CMV) [107]. From this study, it is not clear whether the results were adjusted for confounders, and which ones [107].

Gunji et al. [106], in a well-designed study carried out among 5488 Japanese men (mean age 47± 5 years) and 1906 women (mean age 46±4 years), demonstrated a significant positive relationship between *H. pylori* seropositivity (according to the presence of IgG antibodies) and metabolic syndrome (based on the Japanese diagnostic criteria); adjusted OR: 1.39 (95% CI: 1.18–1.62) Pv<0.001 [106]. This association was independent of known risk factors for metabolic syndrome namely age, sex, diet and smoking [106].

While there is a growing compelling evidence from large epidemiological studies supporting the existence of a positive association between *H. pylori* infection and metabolic syndrome, other studies reported no signification association [108] or reported small magnitude association measures [109]. Therefore, the question of whether *H. pylori* infection is associated with metabolic syndrome, although biologically plausible, remains to be determined, as well as the source of variation among the studies in their findings. Multi-national studies employing similar clinical, epidemiological and diagnostic protocols and methods will be needed to assess true population-to-population variations.

## 6. Conclusions and future directions

Current evidence is conflicting regarding the question of whether *H. pylori* may be associated with an increased risk of DM, metabolic syndrome and poor glycemic control. Although an association between *H. pylori* infection and DM is biologically plausible [110], the nature of such an association is not yet understood. This is due, in part, to important methodological limitations apparent in studies that addressed the relationship between *H. pylori* infection and DM, including inadequate control for socioeconomic status and for known DM risk factors. Moreover, most studies focused on DM, and less on the reversible conditions of IGT, and IFG. Understanding the role in this association of pathogen-related factors, i.e., virulence antigens such as CagA and VacA is still limited. In addition, it is not clear which biological mechanisms may contribute to the postulated excess risk of DM and/or metabolic syndrome in *H. pylori* infected persons compared with uninfected ones. Importantly, it is not yet clear whether *H. pylori* eradication may be beneficial for glycemic control in diabetic patients. Randomized placebo-controlled trials assessing such research questions are lacking.

Addressing these research questions is of great public health and clinical significance given the high prevalence of *H. pylori* infection and significant burden of DM. If *H. pylori* infection is truly involved in the etiology of DM, even to a small magnitude (i.e., small relative risks), the public health impact is expected to be great, given the high prevalence of the infection.

## Author details

Saeda Haj, Michal Raviv and Khitam Muhsen*

*Address all correspondence to: kmuhsen@post.tau.ac.il; khitam15@yahoo.com

Department of Epidemiology and Preventive Medicine, School of Public Health, Sackler Faculty of Medicine, Tel Aviv University, Ramat Aviv, Tel Aviv, Israel

## References

[1] Muhsen K, Jurban M, Goren S, Cohen D. Incidence, age of acquisition and risk factors of Helicobacter pylori infection among Israeli Arab Infants. *J Trop Pediatr* 2012; 58(3): 208–13.

[2] Rothenbacher D, Inceoglu J, Bode G, Brenner H. Acquisition of Helicobacter pylori infection in a high-risk population occurs within the first 2 years of life. *J Pediatr* 2000; 136(6): 744–8.

[3] Torres J, Perez-Perez G, Goodman KJ, et al. A comprehensive review of the natural history of Helicobacter pylori infection in children. *Arch Med Res* 2000; 31(5): 431–69.

[4] Muhsen K, Athamna A, Athamna M, Spungin-Bialik A, Cohen D. Prevalence and risk factors of Helicobacter pylori infection among healthy 3- to 5-year-old Israeli Arab children. *Epidemiol Infect* 2006; 134(5): 990–6.

[5] Muhsen K, Athamna A, Bialik A, Alpert G, Cohen D. Presence of Helicobacter pylori in a sibling is associated with a long-term increased risk of H. pylori infection in Israeli Arab children. *Helicobacter* 2010; 15(2): 108–13.

[6] Weyermann M, Adler G, Brenner H, Rothenbacher D. The mother as source of Helicobacter pylori infection. *Epidemiology* 2006; 17(3): 332–4.

[7] Suerbaum S, Michetti P. Helicobacter pylori infection. *N Engl J Med* 2002; 347(15): 1175–86.

[8] Malfertheiner P, Megraud F, O'Morain CA, et al. Management of Helicobacter pylori infection—the Maastricht IV/Florence Consensus Report. *Gut* 2012; 61(5): 646–64.

[9] Atherton JC. The pathogenesis of Helicobacter pylori-induced gastro-duodenal diseases. *Ann Rev Pathol* 2006; 1: 63–96.

[10] Atherton JC, Blaser MJ. Coadaptation of Helicobacter pylori and humans: ancient history, modern implications. *J Clin Invest* 2009; 119(9): 2475–87.

[11] Kuipers EJ, Uyterlinde AM, Pena AS, et al. Long-term sequelae of Helicobacter pylori gastritis. *Lancet* 1995; 345(8964): 1525–8.

[12] Valle J, Kekki M, Sipponen P, Ihamaki T, Siurala M. Long-term course and consequences of Helicobacter pylori gastritis. Results of a 32-year follow-up study. *Scand J Gastroenterol* 1996; 31(6): 546–50.

[13] Correa P, Haenszel W, Cuello C, et al. Gastric precancerous process in a high risk population: cohort follow-up. *Cancer Res* 1990; 50(15): 4737–40.

[14] Ganga-Zandzou PS, Michaud L, Vincent P, et al. Natural outcome of Helicobacter pylori infection in asymptomatic children: a two-year follow-up study. *Pediatrics* 1999; 104(2 Pt 1): 216–21.

[15] Monack DM, Mueller A, Falkow S. Persistent bacterial infections: the interface of the pathogen and the host immune system. *Na Rev Microbiol* 2004; 2(9): 747–65.

[16] Nomura AM, Kolonel LN, Miki K, et al. Helicobacter pylori, pepsinogen, and gastric adenocarcinoma in Hawaii. *J Infect Dis* 2005; 191(12): 2075–81.

[17] Peek RM, Jr., Blaser MJ. Pathophysiology of Helicobacter pylori-induced gastritis and peptic ulcer disease. *Am J Med* 1997; 102(2): 200–7.

[18] Gao L, Michel A, Weck MN, Arndt V, Pawlita M, Brenner H. Helicobacter pylori infection and gastric cancer risk: evaluation of 15 H. pylori proteins determined by novel multiplex serology. *Cancer Res* 2009; 69(15): 6164–70.

[19] Gao L, Weck MN, Michel A, Pawlita M, Brenner H. Association between chronic atrophic gastritis and serum antibodies to 15 Helicobacter pylori proteins measured by multiplex serology. *Cancer Res* 2009; 69(7): 2973–80.

[20] Epplein M, Zheng W, Xiang YB, et al. Prospective study of Helicobacter pylori biomarkers for gastric cancer risk among Chinese men. *Cancer Epidem Biomar* 2012; 21(12): 2185–92.

[21] Epplein M, Zheng W, Li HL, et al. Diet, Helicobacter pylori strain-specific infection, and gastric cancer risk among Chinese men. *Nutr Cancer* 2014; 66(4): 550–7.

[22] Franceschi F, Gasbarrini A, Polyzos SA, Kountouras J. Extragastric diseases and Helicobacter pylori. *Helicobacter* 2015; 20(Suppl 1): 40–6.

[23] Lai CY, Yang TY, Lin CL, Kao CH. Helicobacter pylori infection and the risk of acute coronary syndrome: a nationwide retrospective cohort study. *Eur J Clin Microbiol Infect Dis* 2015; 34(1): 69–74.

[24] Liu J, Wang F, Shi SL. Helicobacter pylori infection increase the risk of myocardial infarction: a meta-analysis of 26 studies involving more than 20,000 participants. *Helicobacter* 2015; 20(3): 176–83.

[25] Shmuely H, Wattad M, Solodky A, Yahav J, Samra Z, Zafrir N. Association of Helicobacter pylori with coronary artery disease and myocardial infarction assessed by myocardial perfusion imaging. *Isr Med Assoc J* 2014; 16(6): 341–6.

[26] Kountouras J, Tsolaki M, Boziki M, et al. Association between Helicobacter pylori infection and mild cognitive impairment. *Eur J Neurol* 2007; 14(9): 976–82.

[27] Kountouras J, Tsolaki M, Gavalas E, et al. Relationship between Helicobacter pylori infection and Alzheimer disease. *Neurology* 2006; 66(6): 938–40.

[28] Huang WS, Yang TY, Shen WC, Lin CL, Lin MC, Kao CH. Association between Helicobacter pylori infection and dementia. *J Clin Neurosci* 2014; 21(8): 1355–8.

[29] Wang F, Liu J, Lv Z. Association of Helicobacter pylori infection with diabetes mellitus and diabetic nephropathy: a meta-analysis of 39 studies involving more than 20,000 participants. *Scand J Infect Dis* 2013; 45(12): 930–8.

[30] Jeon CY, Haan MN, Cheng C, et al. Helicobacter pylori infection is associated with an increased rate of diabetes. *Diabetes Care* 2012; 35(3): 520–5.

[31] Cover TL, Blaser MJ. Helicobacter pylori in health and disease. *Gastroenterology* 2009; 136(6): 1863–73.

[32] Calam J, Gibbons A, Healey ZV, Bliss P, Arebi N. How does Helicobacter pylori cause mucosal damage? Its effect on acid and gastrin physiology. *Gastroenterology* 1997; 113(6): S43–9.

[33] Sipponen P, Kekki M, Seppala K, Siurala M. The relationships between chronic gastritis and gastric acid secretion. *Aliment Pharmacol Ther* 1996; 10(Suppl 1): 103–18.

[34] Zhang ZW, Patchett SE, Perrett D, Katelaris PH, Domizio P, Farthing MJG. The relation between gastric vitamin C concentrations, mucosal histology, and CagA seropositivity in the human stomach. *Gut* 1998; 43(3): 322–6.

[35] Samloff IM. Cellular localization of group I pepsinogens in human gastric mucosa by immunofluorescence. *Gastroenterology* 1971; 61(2): 185–8.

[36] Samloff IM, Liebman WM. Cellular localization of the group II pepsinogens in human stomach and duodenum by immunofluorescence. *Gastroenterology* 1973; 65(1): 36–42.

[37] Miki K, Urita Y. Using serum pepsinogens wisely in a clinical practice. *J Dig Dis* 2007; 8(1): 8–14.

[38] Graham DY, Nurgalieva ZZ, El-Zimaity HM, et al. Noninvasive versus histologic detection of gastric atrophy in a Hispanic population in North America. *Clin Gastroenterol Hepatol* 2006; 4(3): 306–14.

[39] Song HJ, Jang SJ, Yun SC, et al. Low levels of Pepsinogen I and Pepsinogen I/II ratio are valuable serologic markers for predicting extensive gastric corpus atrophy in patients undergoing endoscopic mucosectomy. *Gut Liver* 2010; 4(4): 475–80.

[40] He CY, Sun LP, Gong YH, Xu Q, Dong NN, Yuan Y. Serum pepsinogen II: a neglected but useful biomarker to differentiate between diseased and normal stomachs. *J Gastroenterol Hepatol* 2011; 26(6): 1039–46.

[41] Roper J, Francois F, Shue PL, et al. Leptin and ghrelin in relation to Helicobacter pylori status in adult males. *J Clin Endocrinol Metab* 2008; 93(6): 2350–7.

[42] Nweneka CV, Prentice AM. Helicobacter pylori infection and circulating ghrelin levels—a systematic review. *BMC Gastroenterol* 2011; 11: 7.

[43] Breidert M, Miehlke S, Glasow A, et al. Leptin and its receptor in normal human gastric mucosa and in Helicobacter pylori-associated gastritis. *Scand J Gastroenterol* 1999; 34(10): 954–61.

[44] Isomoto H, Ueno H, Nishi Y, Wen CY, Nakazato M, Kohno S. Impact of Helicobacter pylori infection on ghrelin and various neuroendocrine hormones in plasma. *World J Gastroenterol* 2005; 11(11): 1644–8.

[45] Francois F, Roper J, Joseph N, et al. The effect of H. pylori eradication on meal-associated changes in plasma ghrelin and leptin. *BMC Gastroenterol* 2011; 11: 37.

[46] Chuang CH, Sheu BS, Yang HB, et al. Gender difference of circulating ghrelin and leptin concentrations in chronic Helicobacter pylori infection. *Helicobacter* 2009; 14(1): 54–60.

[47] Azuma T, Suto H, Ito Y, et al. Gastric leptin and Helicobacter pylori infection. *Gut* 2001; 49(3): 324–9.

[48] Cummings DE, Overduin J. Gastrointestinal regulation of food intake. *J Clin Invest* 2007; 117(1): 13–23.

[49] Kojima M, Hosoda H, Date Y, Nakazato M, Matsuo H, Kangawa K. Ghrelin is a growth-hormone-releasing acylated peptide from stomach. *Nature* 1999; 402(6762): 656–60.

[50] Nakazato M, Murakami N, Date Y, et al. A role for ghrelin in the central regulation of feeding. *Nature* 2001; 409(6817): 194–8.

[51] Bado A, Levasseur S, Attoub S, et al. The stomach is a source of leptin. *Nature* 1998; 394(6695): 790–3.

[52] Jun DW, Lee OY, Lee YY, Choi HS, Kim TH, Yoon BC. Correlation between gastrointestinal symptoms and gastric leptin and ghrelin expression in patients with gastritis. *Digest Dis Sci* 2007; 52(10): 2866–72.

[53] Nishi Y, Isomoto H, Uotani S, et al. Enhanced production of leptin in gastric fundic mucosa with Helicobacter pylori infection. *World J Gastroenterol* 2005; 11(5): 695–9.

[54] Jang EJ, Park SW, Park JS, et al. The influence of the eradication of Helicobacter pylori on gastric ghrelin, appetite, and body mass index in patients with peptic ulcer disease. *J Gastroenterol Hepatol* 2008; 23(Suppl 2): S278–85.

[55] Powers AC. Harrison's Principles of Internal Medicine, 18e. In: Longo DL, Fauci AS, Kasper DL, Hauser SL, Jameson JL, Loscalzo J, editors. Chapter 344, Diabetes Mellitus. 18e ed: The McGraw-Hill Companies, Inc.; 2013.

[56] van Dieren S, Beulens JW, van der Schouw YT, Grobbee DE, Neal B. The global burden of diabetes and its complications: an emerging pandemic. *Eur J Cardiovasc Prev Rehabil* 2010; 17(Suppl 1): S3–8.

[57] Monesi L, Baviera M, Marzona I, et al. Prevalence, incidence and mortality of diagnosed diabetes: evidence from an Italian population-based study. *Diabet Med* 2012; 29(3): 385–92.

[58] Astrup A. Healthy lifestyles in Europe: prevention of obesity and type II diabetes by diet and physical activity. *Public Health Nutr* 2001; 4(2B): 499–515.

[59] Joshi SR, Saboo B, Vadivale M, et al. Prevalence of Diagnosed and Undiagnosed Diabetes and Hypertension in India-Results from the Screening India's Twin Epidemic (SITE) Study. *Diabetes Technol The* 2012; 14(1): 8–15.

[60] Gujral UP, Pradeepa R, Weber MB, Narayan KM, Mohan V. Type 2 diabetes in South Asians: similarities and differences with white Caucasian and other populations. *Ann N Y Acad Sci* 2013; 1281: 51–63.

[61] Steyn NP, Mann J, Bennett PH, et al. Diet, nutrition and the prevention of type 2 diabetes. *Public Health Nutr* 2004; 7(1A): 147–65.

[62] Hu FB, Li TY, Colditz GA, Willett WC, Manson JE. Television watching and other sedentary behaviors in relation to risk of obesity and type 2 diabetes mellitus in women. *JAMA* 2003; 289(14): 1785–91.

[63] Hu FB, Manson JE, Stampfer MJ, et al. Diet, lifestyle, and the risk of type 2 diabetes mellitus in women. *N Engl J Med* 2001; 345(11): 790–7.

[64] Medalie JH, Papier CM, Goldbourt U, Herman JB. Major factors in the development of diabetes mellitus in 10,000 men. *Arch Intern Med* 1975; 135(6): 811–7.

[65] Beaty TH, Neel JV, Fajans SS. Identifying risk factors for diabetes in first degree relatives of non-insulin dependent diabetic patients. *Am J Epidemiol*1982; 115(3): 380–97.

[66] Kadowaki T, Miyake Y, Hagura R, et al. Risk factors for worsening to diabetes in subjects with impaired glucose tolerance. *Diabetologia* 1984; 26(1): 44–9.

[67] van Dam RM. The epidemiology of lifestyle and risk for type 2 diabetes. *Eur J Epidemiol* 2003; 18(12): 1115–25.

[68] Espelt A, Arriola L, Borrell C, Larranaga I, Sandin M, Escolar-Pujolar A. Socioeconomic position and type 2 diabetes mellitus in Europe 1999–2009: a panorama of inequalities. *Current Diabetes Rev* 2011; 7(3): 148–58.

[69] Agardh E, Allebeck P, Hallqvist J, Moradi T, Sidorchuk A. Type 2 diabetes incidence and socio-economic position: a systematic review and meta-analysis. *Int J Epidemiol* 2011; 40(3): 804–18.

[70] Eriksson KF, Lindgarde F. Prevention of type 2 (non-insulin-dependent) diabetes mellitus by diet and physical exercise. The 6-year Malmo feasibility study. *Diabetologia* 1991; 34(12): 891–8.

[71] Ryan DH, Diabetes Prevention Program Research G. Diet and exercise in the prevention of diabetes. *Int J Clin Pract Supplement* 2003; (134): 28–35.

[72] Walker KZ, O'Dea K, Gomez M, Girgis S, Colagiuri R. Diet and exercise in the prevention of diabetes. *J Hum Nutr Diet* 2010; 23(4): 344–52.

[73] Sukala WR, Page R, Cheema BS. Exercise training in high-risk ethnic populations with type 2 diabetes: a systematic review of clinical trials. *Diabetes Res Clin Pr* 2012; 97(2): 206–16.

[74] Weigt J, Malfertheiner P. Influence of Helicobacter pylori on gastric regulation of food intake. *Curr Opin Clin Nutr Metab Care* 2009; 12(5): 522–5.

[75] Isomoto H, Ueno H, Saenko VA, et al. Impact of Helicobacter pylori infection on gastric and plasma ghrelin dynamics in humans. *Am J Gastroenterol* 2005; 100(8): 1711–20.

[76] Liew PL, Lee WJ, Lee YC, Chen WY. Gastric ghrelin expression associated with Helicobacter pylori infection and chronic gastritis in obese patients. *Obes Surg* 2006; 16(5): 612–9.

[77] Cummings DE, Purnell JQ, Frayo RS, Schmidova K, Wisse BE, Weigle DS. A preprandial rise in plasma ghrelin levels suggests a role in meal initiation in humans. *Diabetes* 2001; 50(8): 1714–9.

[78] Shintani M, Ogawa Y, Ebihara K, et al. Ghrelin, an endogenous growth hormone secretagogue, is a novel orexigenic peptide that antagonizes leptin action through the activation of hypothalamic neuropeptide Y/Y1 receptor pathway. *Diabetes* 2001; 50(2): 227–32.

[79] Wolf G. Leptin: the weight-reducing plasma protein encoded by the obese gene. *Nutr Rev* 1996; 54(3): 91–3.

[80] Halaas JL, Gajiwala KS, Maffei M, et al. Weight-reducing effects of the plasma protein encoded by the obese gene. *Science* 1995; 269(5223): 543–6.

[81] Chen Y, Blaser MJ. Association between gastric Helicobacter pylori colonization and glycated hemoglobin levels. *J Infect Dis* 2012; 205(8): 1195–202.

[82] Polyzos SA, Kountouras J, Zavos C, Deretzi G. The association between Helicobacter pylori infection and insulin resistance: a systematic review. *Helicobacter* 2011; 16(2): 79–88.

[83] Bener A, Micallef R, Afifi M, Derbala M, Al-Mulla HM, Usmani MA. Association between type 2 diabetes mellitus and Helicobacter pylori infection. *Turk J Gastroenterol* 2007; 18(4): 225–9.

[84] Zhou X, Zhang C, Wu J, Zhang G. Association between Helicobacter pylori infection and diabetes mellitus: a meta-analysis of observational studies. *Diabetes Res Clin Pract* 2013; 99(2): 200–8.

[85] Wang F, Liu J, Lv Z. Association of Helicobacter pylori infection with diabetes mellitus and diabetic nephropathy: a meta-analysis of 39 studies involving more than 20,000 participants. *Scand J Infect Dis* 2013; 45(12): 930–8.

[86] Hsieh MC, Wang SSW, Hsieh YT, Kuo FC, Soon MS, Wu DC. Helicobacter pylori infection associated with high HbA1c and type 2 diabetes. *Eur J Clin Invest* 2013; 43(9): 949–56.

[87] Dore MP, Bilotta M, Malaty HM, et al. Diabetes mellitus and Helicobacter pylori infection. *Nutrition* 2000; 16(6): 407–10.

[88] Lutsey PL, Pankow JS, Bertoni AG, Szklo M, Folsom AR. Serological evidence of infections and type 2 diabetes: the MultiEthnic Study of Atherosclerosis. *Diabet Med* 2009; 26(2): 149–52.

[89] Xia HH, Talley NJ, Kam EP, Young LJ, Hammer J, Horowitz M. Helicobacter pylori infection is not associated with diabetes mellitus, nor with upper gastrointestinal symptoms in diabetes mellitus. *Am J Gastroenterol* 2001; 96(4): 1039–46.

[90] Demir M, Gokturk HS, Ozturk NA, Kulaksizoglu M, Serin E, Yilmaz U. Helicobacter pylori prevalence in diabetes mellitus patients with dyspeptic symptoms and its relationship to glycemic control and late complications. *Dig Dis Sci* 2008; 53(10): 2646–9.

[91] Longo-Mbenza B, Nsenga JN, Mokondjimobe E, et al. Helicobacter pylori infection is identified as a cardiovascular risk factor in Central Africans. *VascHealth Risk manag* 2012; 6: 455–61.

[92] Cenerelli S, Bonazzi P, Galeazzi R, et al. Helicobacter pylori masks differences in homocysteine plasma levels between controls and type 2 diabetic patients. *Eur J Clin Invest* 2002; 32(3): 158–62.

[93] Horikawa C, Kodama S, Fujihara K, et al. Association of Helicobacter pylori infection with glycemic control in patients with diabetes: a meta-analysis. *J Diabetes Res* 2014.

[94] Dai YN, Yu WL, Zhu HT, Ding JX, Yu CH, Li YM. Is Helicobacter pylori infection associated with glycemic control in diabetics? *World J Gastroenterol* 2015; 21(17): 5407–16.

[95] Zojaji H, Ataei E, Sherafat SJ, Ghobakhlou M, Fatemi SR. The effect of the treatment of helicobacter pylori infection on the glycemic control in type 2 diabetes mellitus. *Gastroenterol Hepatol* 2013; 6(1): 36–40.

[96] Wada Y, Hamamoto Y, Kawasaki Y, et al. The eradication of Helicobacter pylori does not affect glycemic control in Japanese subjects with type 2 diabetes. *Jap Clin Med* 2013; 4: 41–3.

[97] Vafaeimanesh J, Rajabzadeh R, Ahmadi A, et al. Effect of Helicobacter pylori eradication on glycaemia control in patients with type 2 diabetes mellitus and comparison of two therapeutic regimens. *Arab J Gastroenterol* 2013; 14(2): 55–8.

[98] Akanuma M, Yanai A, Sakamoto K, et al. Influence of Helicobacter pylori eradication on the management of type 2 diabetes. *Hepato-Gastroenterology* 2012; 59(114): 641–5.

[99] Candelli M, Rigante D, Marietti G, et al. Helicobacter pylori eradication rate and glycemic control in young patients with type 1 diabetes. *J Pediatr Gastroenterol Nutr* 2004; 38(4): 422–5.

[100] Begue RE, Gomez R, Compton T, Vargas A. Effect of Helicobacter pylori eradication in the glycemia of children with type 1 diabetes: a preliminary study. *South Med J* 2002; 95(8): 842–5.

[101] de Luis DA, Cordero JM, Caballero C, et al. Effect of the treatment of Helicobacter pylori infection on gastric emptying and its influence on the glycaemic control in type 1 diabetes mellitus. *DiabResClin Pract* 2001; 52(1): 1–9.

[102] Grundy SM, Cleeman JI, Daniels SR, et al. Diagnosis and management of the metabolic syndrome: an American Heart Association/National Heart, Lung, and Blood Institute scientific statement. *Curr Opin Cardiol* 2006; 21(1): 1–6.

[103] Grundy SM, Cleeman JI, Daniels SR, et al. Diagnosis and management of the metabolic syndrome: an American Heart Association/National Heart, Lung, and Blood Institute Scientific Statement. *Circulation* 2005; 112(17): 2735–52.

[104] Polyzos SA, Kountouras J. Novel advances in the association between helicobacter pylori infection, metabolic syndrome, and related morbidity. *Helicobacter* 2015; 20(6): 405–9.

[105] Chen TP, Hung HF, Chen MK, et al. Helicobacter pylori infection is positively associated with metabolic syndrome in Taiwanese adults: a cross-sectional study. *Helicobacter* 2015; 20(3): 184–91.

[106] Gunji T, Matsuhashi N, Sato H, et al. Helicobacter pylori infection is significantly associated with metabolic syndrome in the Japanese population. *Am J Gastroenterol* 2008; 103(12): 3005–10.

[107] Nabipour I, Vahdat K, Jafari SM, Pazoki R, Sanjdideh Z. The association of metabolic syndrome and Chlamydia pneumoniae, Helicobacter pylori, cytomegalovirus, and herpes simplex virus type 1: The Persian Gulf Healthy Heart Study. *Cardiovascr Diabetol* 2006; 5.

[108] Naja F, Nasreddine L, Hwalla N, et al. Association of H. pylori infection with insulin resistance and metabolic syndrome among Lebanese adults. *Helicobacter* 2012; 17(6): 444–51.

[109] Shin DW, Kwon HT, Kang JM, et al. Association between metabolic syndrome and Helicobacter pylori infection diagnosed by histologic status and serological status. *J Clin Gastroenterol* 2012; 46(10): 840–5.

[110] He C, Yang Z, Lu NH. Helicobacter pylori infection and diabetes: is it a myth or fact? *World J Gastroenterol* 2014; 20(16): 4607–17.

[111] El-Eshmawy MM, El-Hawary AK, Abdel Gawad SS, El-Baiomy AA. Helicobacter pylori infection might be responsible for the interconnection between type 1 diabetes and autoimmune thyroiditis. *Diabetol* Metab Syndr 2011; 3(1).

[112] Colombo C TP, Meloni GF, Marinaro AM, Ogana A, Meloni T. Seroprevalence of Helicobacter pylori in children with type 1 diabetes mellitus in Sardinia. Diabetes Nutr Metab 2002; 15: 91–5.